From the Editors of

Health®

The

Carb Lovers DIET

COOK BOOK

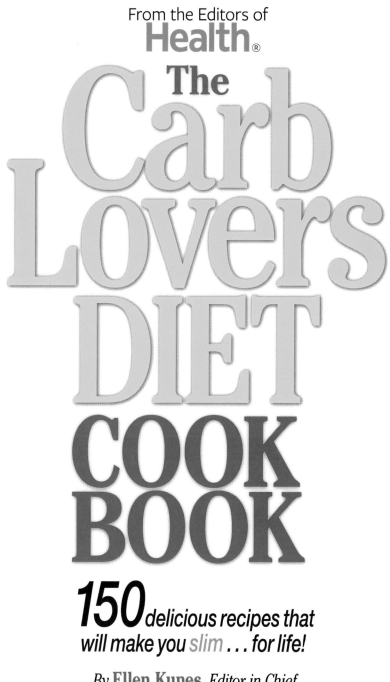

150 *delicious recipes that will make you slim . . . for life!*

By **Ellen Kunes**, *Editor in Chief,*
and **Frances Largeman-Roth**, *RD*
Health *magazine*

OXMOOR HOUSE®

ISBN-13: 978-0-8487-3477-0
ISBN-10: 0-8487-3477-7
Library of Congress Control Number: 2011936985
Printed in the United States of America
First Printing 2011

This book is intended as a general reference only, and is not to be used as a substitute for medical
advice or treatment. We urge you to consult your physician regarding any individual
medical conditions or specific health-related issues or questions.

Health
Editor-in-Chief: Ellen Kunes
Creative Director: Ben Margherita
Managing Editor: Marc Einsele
Food and Nutrition Director: Frances Largeman-Roth, RD
Health.com Editor-in-Chief: Amy O'Connor

Art Department
Design Director: Trish McGinty-Boyles
Art Directors: Robin Brown, Robin Helman

Photo
Photo Director: Jo Miller
Senior Photo Editor: Tara Canova
Art and Production Intern: Molly McGaughey

Copy and Research
Copy Chief: Marti Trgovich
Contributing Copy Editors: Jamie Beckman, Christopher Jagger
Research Editor: Michael Gollust
Researchers: Sarah DiGiulio, Carina Storrs

Production
Production Designer: Ramón A. Gamarra

Test Kitchen and Diet Plans
Adeena Sussman
Caroline Wright
Sarah Abrams
Sonthe Burge, RD
Kate Slate

Dedication

Ellen

For my mom, who taught me how to cook, and
for my dad, who loved carbs—especially the
chocolate kind!—and enjoyed them every single day.

Frances

For my mother, who taught me the importance of
hearty bread and a well-balanced meal. And for
my wonderful husband, Jon, and sweet kids, Willa
and Leo—thanks for all your love and support.

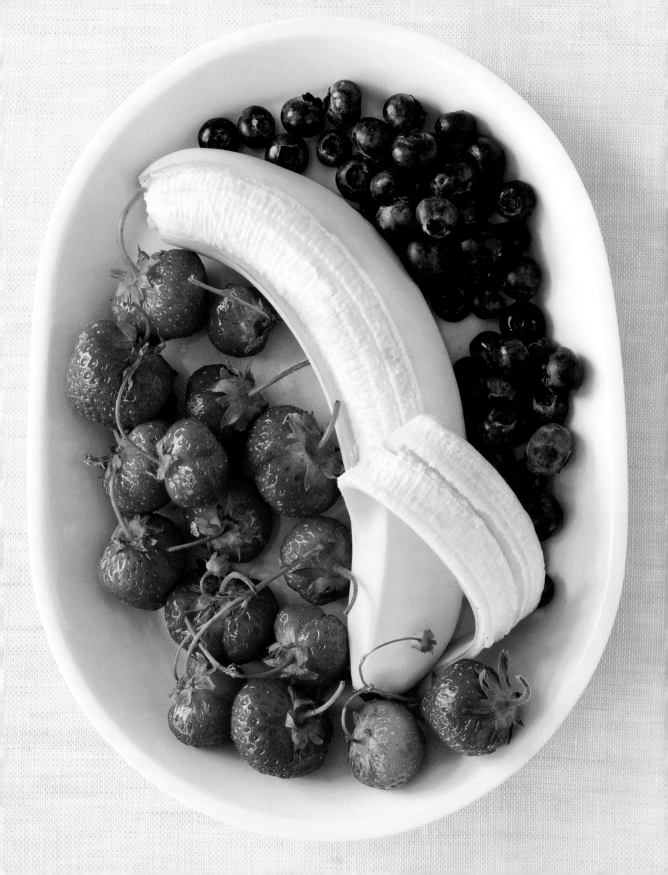

Contents

Acknowledgments

The CarbLovers Diet Cookbook is the culmination of years of researching how we all can achieve our weight-loss goals while still enjoying our favorite foods. But it's also my personal favorite in the *CarbLovers* series, which includes *The CarbLovers Diet Pocket Guide* and the original *CarbLovers Diet* book. I know *Health* and Health.com's audience of nearly 19 million will love the easy, delicious recipes, smart advice, and stunning photography as much as I do. Lots of credit goes to my dedicated and talented team, especially my co-author and *Health*'s food and nutrition director, Frances Largeman-Roth, RD, as well as Marc Einsele, Amy O'Connor, Trish McGinty-Boyles, Sarah DiGiulio, and Michael Gollust, who worked on *The CarbLovers Diet Cookbook* while putting out a great magazine and website. Thanks also to Sonthe Burge, RD— a tireless resource and advocate for *CarbLovers* dieters—and copy editor Christopher Jagger.

We also want to thank everyone at Time Home Entertainment Inc. and Oxmoor House, especially Richard Fraiman, Jim Childs, Vanessa Tiongson, and Helen Wan.

We'd also like to thank Adeena Sussman, Caroline Wright, Sarah Abrams, and Kate Slate for their culinary creativity and nutrition wisdom. Special appreciation goes to Andrew McCaul, Stephana Bottom, Jo Miller, and Alistair Turnbull for the absolutely gorgeous photography in this book, which will inspire all to make these great dishes. And a big shout-out to our celebrity chefs— Guy Fieri, Wolfgang Puck, Cat Cora, Carla Hall, Michael Chiarello, Donatella Arpaia, Emily Luchetti, Candice Kumai, Cristina Ferrare, Joe Bastianich, Gail Simmons, Allysa Torey, Matt Lewis, and Renato Poliafito—for their incredible generosity and amazing carb-filled recipes!

Finally, our deepest gratitude goes to those who enjoyed *The CarbLovers Diet* and asked for more recipes and menus. This book is for all of you!

Ellen Kunes,
Editor-in-Chief, *Health* magazine

PART 1
Cooking the CarbLovers Way

Cooking with CarbLovers!

"A diet rich in carbs is the best way to get and stay slim." Believe it or not, that was a controversial statement when it first appeared in *The CarbLovers Diet* just over a year ago. Many were skeptical of the promise of a weight-loss plan based on delicious pasta, pizza, and baked potatoes. (To be honest, even we couldn't predict how well it would work!)

We did, however, have faith in the scientific evidence that eating the right carbs would help dieters—even those who failed on other plans—stay slim for life, without ever feeling deprived. And we were excited about encouraging people to eat more foods that contain Resistant Starch, the star ingredient of *The CarbLovers Diet*.

Nearly 200 studies have shown Resistant Starch, found naturally in whole grains, potatoes, beans, and some fruits, to be an extraordinary weight-loss tool. It's 100 percent safe, and it acts as a powerful appetite suppressant and metabolism booster.

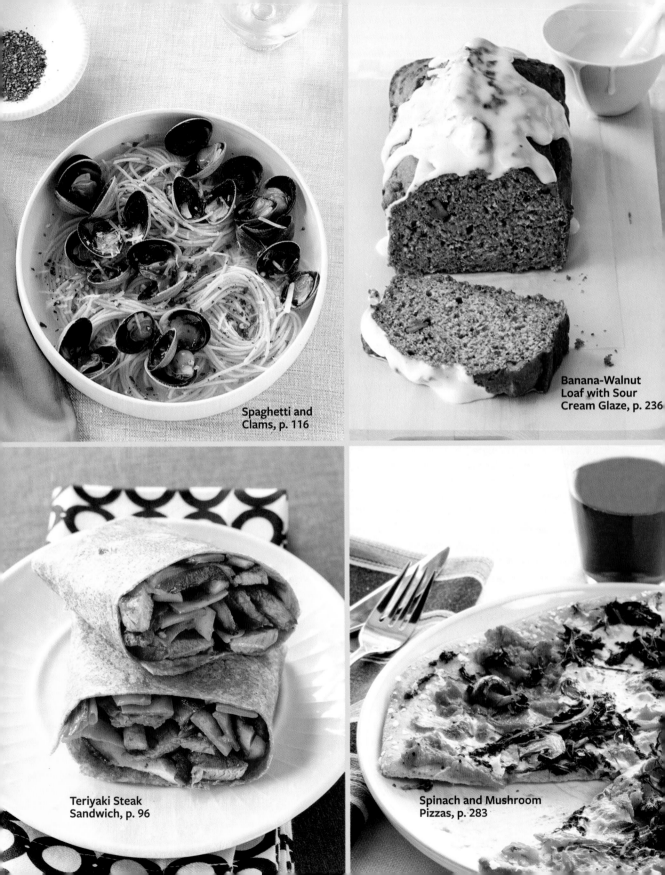

Spaghetti and
Clams, p. 116

Banana-Walnut
Loaf with Sour
Cream Glaze, p. 236

Teriyaki Steak
Sandwich, p. 96

Spinach and Mushroom
Pizzas, p. 283

Today it seems like everyone is talking about Resistant Starch, but not because of a bunch of studies. That carbs make you slim, not heavy, is practically common knowledge, thanks to the incredible success of *The CarbLovers Diet*. The first book spent an amazing nine weeks on *The New York Times* best-seller list, spun off a wildly successful app and *The CarbLovers Diet Pocket Guide*, and generated national media attention. *CarbLovers Diet* fans now include celebrities, renowned chefs, and top doctors and researchers. *CarbLovers* even has its own dedicated communities on Facebook and Twitter.

CarbLovers dieters loved the delicious recipes, meal plans anyone can stick to, and easy substitutes and grab-and-go food items. But you told us you wanted more—much more. A breakthrough diet plan that's even simpler to follow. More information about finding and cooking foods with Resistant Starch, the super carb that fills you up and melts fat. More advice for adapting *CarbLovers* to your lifestyle. More drink suggestions—including cocktails. More ideas for following the *CarbLovers Diet* on vacation, during the holidays, with your family, and when you're on the go. More cooking tips. And, most of all, you wanted a whole lot more recipes!

The CarbLovers Diet Cookbook delivers. The Recipe Collection features 150 new, quick and easy, totally yummy recipes—including updated versions of your favorite *CarbLovers* comfort foods. You won't believe what we've cooked up!

In *The CarbLovers Diet Cookbook*, you'll enjoy hearty buckwheat crepes (page 62) or moist, rich banana bread (page 59) for breakfast; decadent Cobb salad (page 182) or silky butternut squash soup (page 80) for lunch; and a succulent spice-rubbed pork loin (page 151) or shrimp tacos (page 148) for dinner. You can even make holiday cookies (page 289) or throw a cocktail party (page 312) with our special-occasion menus, which make entertaining a snap.

As a bonus, we're thrilled to offer you custom recipes from your favorite carb-loving celebrity chefs, including Guy Fieri, Wolfgang Puck, and Cat Cora!

The CarbLovers Diet Cookbook has been created by the same food and nutrition experts who developed the original *CarbLovers*, with a new, proven diet plan and recipes so delicious you'll want to serve them to company. So go ahead: Enjoy our amazing new carb-filled meals!

Ellen Kunes,
Editor in Chief, *Health* magazine

How Carbs Make You Thin...For Life

I'm guessing you're digging into this book for one of two (really good) reasons: 1) You lost weight on *The CarbLovers Diet* and want more delicious, easy, carb-rich recipes; or 2) You just love great food—especially dishes bursting with delicious carbs. Learning that your favorite pasta, pizza, and potato dishes will actually help you lose weight has made you hungry for more details.

The best news: The research behind *The CarbLovers Diet Cookbook* shows strong evidence that a diet rich in carbs is the healthiest and most effective way to get and stay slim for life. But here's something to keep in mind: These carbs aren't the refined kind, packed with tons of additives and preservatives that come in crinkly packages from a vending machine. *The CarbLovers Diet* isn't about junk food (though you are allowed daily indulgences, including chocolate). The carb-rich foods that make you slender are packed with fiber, antioxidants, and Resistant Starch, the star ingredient that has helped so many feel full and lose weight on *The CarbLovers Diet*.

The CarbLovers Diet's Secret Weapon

What exactly is Resistant Starch? Carbohydrate-rich foods contain two types of starch. One is high-glycemic starch; like sugar, it gets absorbed into the bloodstream quickly and gives you a fast hit of energy. Another is called Resistant Starch, so named because it "resists" digestion. Hundreds of studies have shown Resistant Starch to be a natural appetite suppressant, metabolism booster, and overall health promoter. It produces fatty acids that trigger weight loss by turning on enzymes that melt fat, especially in the abdominal area; encouraging your liver to switch to a fat-burning state; and boosting satiety hormones that make you get and stay full longer. Resistant Starch is more than safe; you really can't eat too much of it. In fact, most people consume too little—about 5 grams a day. Researchers believe we need at least twice that amount for optimal health and weight loss. That's why the *CarbLovers* menus include 10 to 15 grams daily of this important fat-burning nutrient, served up in delicious recipes like our Cornflake-Crusted Chicken Tenders (p. 168) and Triple-Cheese Mac (p. 126).

The Science of Carbs and Health

The CarbLovers Diet Cookbook doesn't hinge solely on the health and weight-loss benefits of Resistant Starch, though. All of our recipes (which start on page 34) have been created to pack the best possible ratio of the nutrients that research shows help to melt fat, boost satiety, and promote good health—and get you a much flatter belly. Belly bloat is one of the key symptoms of constipation, a common side effect of not eating enough healthy carbs.

The amazing carb-filled recipes in this book, including Chicken Cacciatore with Rigatoni (p. 122) and Grilled Flank Steak Fajitas (p. 154), taste just as delicious as they sound. But they also contain a mix of carbohydrates that make them healthier and much more filling than most protein- or fat-loaded foods. The Resistant Starch and fiber in our recipes act as powerful appetite suppressants. They fill you up because they are digested more slowly than other types of foods and trigger a greater sensation of fullness in both your brain and your belly. Eating *The CarbLovers Diet* way, according to research, can help you consume 10 percent fewer calories a day—without ever feeling hungry!

Scientific evidence bears this out. For instance, one groundbreaking study looked at thousands of people to see what factors determine whether they stayed slim or gained weight over time. Conclusion: The slimmest people ate the most good carbs—the kind you'll find in the recipes in this book—and the chubbiest ate the least. The researchers confirmed that your odds of getting and staying slim are best when carbs comprise up to 64 percent of your total calorie intake, which mirrors what a day of eating the *CarbLovers* way delivers.

Another recent study found that making a simple lifestyle switch—such as eating more carbs at dinner—can result in both weight loss and a reduction in body fat. Researchers in Israel put 78 overweight or obese police officers on a diet. Half were given a low-calorie weight-loss plan, while the other group followed the same diet but ate most of their carbohydrates at dinner. Incredibly, after six months the carbs-at-dinner group lost both more weight and body fat—and they reported feeling less hungry than other dieters. The evening carb eaters also got healthier, with improvements in both their blood sugar and cholesterol levels. Researchers believe that eating your carbs at night may help elevate satiety hormones during the day, preventing feelings of hunger. Bottom line: Carbs satisfy, no matter what time of day you eat them.

The CarbLovers Diet may actually be one of the healthiest diets you can follow, whether you're trying to lose weight or simply maintain your current weight. Scores of studies conducted at top research institutions worldwide show that eating the right carbs is one of the smartest preventive measures you can take to keep your heart healthy, your cholesterol and blood pressure low, and your blood sugar balanced. A recent study by researchers in the United Kingdom published in *The American Journal of Clinical Nutrition* found that including three servings of whole grain foods in the diets of healthy people helped significantly lower their blood pressure; the researchers concluded that daily consumption of whole grains could thus decrease the incidence of stroke by 25 percent and coronary artery disease by 15 percent.

How Carbs Make You Happy

As you cook and eat according to *The CarbLovers Diet Cookbook*, you might start to feel calmer, happier, and less stressed. The reason? Carbs boost mood-regulating, stress-reducing chemicals in the brain, while high-protein, fatty foods may deplete them, says Grant Brinkworth, PhD, lead researcher of a study published in the *Archives of Internal Medicine*. He followed 51 dieters on a carb-rich diet and 55 dieters on a low-carb plan. After a year, the carb eaters felt happier, calmer, and more focused than the carb-deprived group, who reported feeling stressed out. Stress produces high levels of hormones, such as cortisol, which boost your appetite and can lead to bingeing, says obesity researcher Elissa Epel, PhD, associate professor in the department of psychiatry at the University of California, San Francisco.

In other words, enjoying the delicious recipes in *The CarbLovers Diet Cookbook* will make you look good and feel great! "Dieters feel so empowered once they lose weight on carbs. For the first time, they are able to lose weight by eating in a balanced manner, without cutting out entire food groups," says Sari Greaves, RD, spokesperson for the American Dietetic Association.

What Foods Contain

FOOD	PORTION	RS
Banana, slightly green	1 medium (7–8″)	12.5
Banana, ripe	1 medium (7–8″)	4.7
Oatmeal, uncooked/toasted	½ cup	4.6
Beans, white, cooked/canned	½ cup	3.8
Lentils, cooked	½ cup	3.4
Potatoes, cooked and cooled*	1 potato, small	3.2
Plantain, cooked	½ cup, slices	2.7
Beans, garbanzo, cooked/canned	½ cup	2.1
Pasta, whole wheat, cooked	1 cup	2.0
Barley, pearl, cooked	½ cup	1.9
Pasta, white, cooked and cooled	1 cup	1.9
Beans, kidney, cooked/canned	½ cup	1.8
Potatoes, boiled (skin and flesh)*	1 potato, small	1.8
Rice, brown, cooked	½ cup	1.7
Beans, pinto, cooked/canned	½ cup	1.6
Peas, canned/frozen	½ cup	1.6
Beans, black, cooked/canned	½ cup	1.5
Millet, cooked	½ cup	1.5

*The Resistant Starch content of potatoes varies depending on cooking method and temperature served.

Resistant Starch?

FOOD	PORTION	RS
Pasta, white, cooked	1 cup	1.5
Potatoes, baked (skin and flesh)*	1 potato, small	1.4
Bread, pumpernickel	1-ounce slice	1.3
Corn polenta, cooked	½ cup	1.0
Potato chips	1 ounce	1.0
Yam, cooked	½ cup, cubes	1.0
Bread, rye (whole)	1-ounce slice	0.9
Cornflakes	1 cup	0.9
Puffed wheat	1¼ cups	0.9
Tortillas, corn	1 ounce, 6" tortilla	0.8
English muffin	1 whole muffin	0.7
Bread, sourdough	1-ounce slice	0.6
Crackers, rye crispbread	2 crispbreads	0.6
Oatmeal, cooked	1 cup	0.5
Bread, Italian	1-ounce slice	0.3
Bread, whole grain	1-ounce slice	0.3
Corn chips	1 ounce	0.2
Crackers, crispbread (melba)	½ cup rounds	0.2

In the Kitchen
With *CarbLovers*

Cooking the *CarbLovers* way is surprisingly easy. It's fun, affordable, and oh-so-satisfying. But don't take our word for it! Dieters who kicked their fast-food and vending-machine habits tell us they feel an incredible sense of accomplishment shopping for the freshest ingredients and cooking at home, then savoring dishes like Chicken Cacciatore with Rigatoni (page 122) and Maple-Glazed Cod with Baby Bok Choy (page 144) on a daily basis. Some even say cooking gives them an edge when it comes to getting and staying slim for life.

Here's why they might be right: The recipes in *The CarbLovers Diet Cookbook* make dieting almost effortless. They take all the guesswork out of counting calories, tallying Resistant Starch, and planning meals. Each is designed to have a specific nutrition profile that allows you to enjoy three full meals a day plus a snack and dessert—while still losing weight. And these recipes are foolproof. We tested each recipe again and again, in real kitchens by real people, so we know they really work!

Read on for details on cooking with *CarbLovers* recipes, plus advice on stocking and organizing your kitchen. Follow our easy tips and soon you'll be cooking the *CarbLovers* way with every meal.

CarbLovers Cooking 101

Beans and Legumes

Many recipes in *The CarbLovers Diet Cookbook* call for beans, and for good reason. Beans are among the healthiest, most slimming, and most affordable foods you can find. Loaded with Resistant Starch, beans and legumes (such as lentils) pack both types of fiber—soluble and insoluble (one fills you up and helps lower cholesterol; the other keeps your digestive system humming along). Getting enough fiber also speeds weight loss: A Brigham Young University study of 252 women found that every extra gram of fiber consumed resulted in half a pound of weight loss. (But you don't have to count grams; *The CarbLovers Diet* makes sure you get the recommended 25–35 grams of fiber every day.)

Beans are incredibly easy to cook with. Canned beans are fine to use, as they pack the same nutritional benefits as dried (rinse and drain them first, to lower the sodium that comes in the canning liquid). But do try cooking beans from scratch, in large batches. This method tends to yield better-tasting and sodium-free beans. (It's also super-cheap!) Cooked beans freeze well in airtight containers and will keep for 6 months or longer. To use, thaw, then toss into salads, soups, even pasta. Beans also make a great base for spreads and dips, such as our Layered Spicy Black Bean and Cheddar Dip (page 208).

STOVETOP BEANS Sort and wash dried beans, discarding any that look shriveled or broken. Rinse in a colander, then soak in fresh, unsalted water in a large bowl for at least 8 hours or overnight. Bonus! Soaking beans cuts down on the complex sugars that can cause gas.

When beans have soaked for at least 8 hours, drain and pour into a large stockpot or Dutch oven. Cover and bring to a boil, then reduce heat and let simmer for 1 to 3 hours or until beans are tender (the larger the beans, the more time they will take to cook). Salting beans before they're cooked makes them tough, so wait to salt until you are ready to serve.

PRESSURE-COOKER BEANS Pressure-cooking beans is a snap. Never fill the cooker more than ⅔ full, and be sure to add a teaspoon of oil to the water to prevent foaming. Use 1 cup of beans to 4 cups water, and check the instructions on your appliance for exact cook times. Cooking time for very dry or large beans will be shorter if you presoak your beans overnight.

TIP:
Small beans and legumes—such as split peas and lentils—cook up quickly, so there's no need to soak or put them in a pressure cooker.

STORAGE Store dried beans at room temperature in an airtight container for up to a year. Just keep them away from sunlight, which may cause their color to fade. Canned beans last up to 5 years. Refrigerate cooked beans for up to a week or freeze for 6 months.

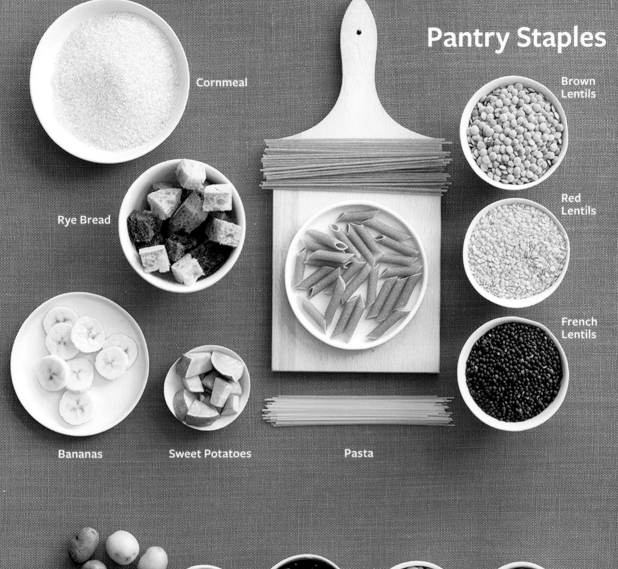

Pantry Staples

Cornmeal

Brown Lentils

Rye Bread

Red Lentils

French Lentils

Bananas

Sweet Potatoes

Pasta

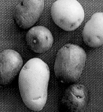

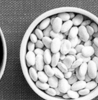

Potatoes

Pinto Beans

Black Beans

Navy Beans

Kidney Beans

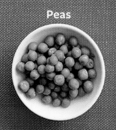
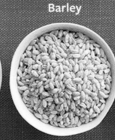
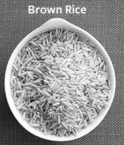

Peas

Rolled Oats

Barley

Brown Rice

Barley

Barley is one of the best grain sources of Resistant Starch and a key source of whole grains in *The CarbLovers Diet*. Barley has a tight-fitting inedible hull as it grows in the field. It's removed through a process called pearling that scrapes away the hull. Unfortunately, some of the bran gets removed too; try barley labeled "hulled" to be sure that your barley has had the hull removed without removing the bran. Pearl barley, the kind found in most grocery stores and used in our recipes, is also very filling and nutritious. Creamy, chewy, with a subtle flavor that combines well with others, pair barley with any sauce or use as a substitute for rice or pasta.

STOVETOP BARLEY Sauté 1 cup dry barley in 1 teaspoon hot oil in a medium saucepan over medium-high heat for 4 minutes or until lightly browned. Stir in 2 cups water. Bring to a boil; cover, reduce heat, and simmer 30–40 minutes or until barley is just tender and slightly chewy. Remove from heat; let stand 5 minutes.

STORAGE Cooked barley can be refrigerated for 3–5 days, or you can freeze it in an airtight container for up to 6 months. Store uncooked barley for 6 months or longer in an airtight container at room temperature.

Rice

Although it takes longer to cook than white or yellow rice, brown rice is worth the time because it's a nutritional powerhouse, packing Resistant Starch, fiber, and other nutrients in every nutty bite. That means it will take longer to digest and you'll feel full for a lot longer.

STOVETOP RICE In a saucepan, combine 1 cup of uncooked brown rice with 2 cups of water (or in any amounts using this 1:2 ratio). Bring the mixture to a boil, stirring occasionally, then reduce heat. Cover and simmer for about 50 minutes, until cooked.

STORAGE Cooked rice can be kept in the refrigerator for up to 5 days. Uncooked rice can last 6 months or longer stored in an airtight container at room temperature.

Pasta

Who doesn't adore pasta? *The CarbLovers Diet Cookbook* offers loads of mouth-watering pasta dishes, including ones from top chefs, like Michael Chiarello's Fusilli Michelangelo with Roasted Chicken (page 270) and Joe Bastianich's Scoglio (page 280). The pasta recipes we developed for this book include traditional "white" pasta, as well as flavorful and nutritious whole-grain pastas. The whole grain variety has double to triple the fiber and more protein than regular pasta, so you'll feel fuller faster and eat less now—and later.

STOVETOP PASTA Bring a large stockpot filled with water to boil. Salt the water once it starts boiling and add the pasta. Stir the pasta gently while cooking to prevent clumping, and cook according to package directions (though you can test for doneness a minute or two earlier). Reserve ½ cup of cooking water to add more flavor and body to your sauce. Drain pasta in a colander.

STORAGE While pasta is best when freshly cooked, you can refrigerate it in an airtight container, with or without sauce for 3 days. Fresh (not dried) pasta can be kept in the refrigerator for up to 1 week or frozen for up to a month. Dried pasta lasts longer—up to 2 years—when stored in a dry, cool place.

Oatmeal

Steel-cut oatmeal, often called Irish oatmeal, is made from whole grain oats that are cracked, not rolled. These whole grains are an amazing source of Resistant Starch, especially when cooked and processed as little as possible. They're also rich in soluble fiber, which absorbs water and helps you feel full, so you get—and stay—trim.

The best way to get your Resistant Starch and fiber from oatmeal is to cook steel-cut oats on your stovetop (rolled and instant oats usually don't have the same health and weight-loss benefits as the whole-grain type). Another way to up your oat intake is to replace half your all-purpose flour with store-bought or homemade oat flour (grind rolled oats in a food processor) for baking cookies, pancakes, and quick breads. You get twice the fiber and fewer calories.

STOVETOP OATMEAL The basic recipe is 1 part oats to 3 parts water. Add both to a saucepan and bring to a boil, then simmer until the liquid is absorbed, about 35 minutes. It's also easy to cook batches of steel-cut oats ahead of time. Before bed, combine 1 cup oats with 3 cups water, bring the mixture to a boil, then turn off the heat. In the morning, simmer for 5–10 minutes until fully cooked. Keep the extra in the freezer or in the fridge until needed, then warm up.

If all you have time to make is rolled oats, go for it—oats are still one of the healthiest grains you can eat. Combine 1 part oats with 2 parts water or low-fat milk. Bring the mixture to a boil, then reduce heat. You will only need to cook these oats for another couple of minutes—don't leave them cooking for much longer, or they'll get mushy.

MICROWAVE OATMEAL Combine ½ cup old-fashioned rolled oats or instant steel-cut oatmeal with 1 cup 1% milk or water in a small microwave-safe bowl. Microwave on HIGH for 3–5 minutes.

STORAGE Cooked oatmeal can be kept in the refrigerator for up to 5 days. Store uncooked oatmeal in an airtight container in a cool, dry place. It can be used for up to 6 months. Some packaged brands of oats last longer—check the packaging before storing.

Potatoes and Sweet Potatoes

TIP:
Do not freeze cooked potatoes, as this can turn them mushy.

Potatoes have gotten a bad rap in the past, but you no longer need an excuse to enjoy your favorite root vegetable. All potatoes are super healthy carbs and a good source of Resistant Starch, especially when cooked and cooled (remember, bringing cooked potatoes to room temperature boosts their Resistant Starch content). They are also a natural source of proteinase inhibitor, a type of protein that may increase levels of satiety hormones and curb hunger. Of course, they're delicious too! That's why baked potatoes, sweet potatoes, mashes of all varieties, yams, baked fries, and even potato chips are allowed on *The CarbLovers Diet*.

Potatoes of every stripe are a dieter's best friend in part because they are incredibly filling. One large baked potato, for instance, will run you fewer than 300 calories. Plus, potatoes are among the richest sources of potassium, the electrolyte that helps to maintain the body's fluid balance (and helps prevent muscle cramps). Sweet potatoes are a great source of beta-carotene; one medium sweet potato packs nearly three times the recommended daily amount. Aside from being rich in potassium, these tasty tubers boast immunity-boosting vitamin C and vitamin B6, key for maintaining a healthy nervous system.

Choose smooth-skinned potatoes and cut out any dark spots with a paring knife or the tip of your peeler (if they've sprouted, throw them out!). If you want to keep the peel on during cooking, check to make sure there is no green tinge to the skin. If there is, simply peel it off.

STORAGE Potatoes keep well for weeks in a cool, dry place, preferably on a countertop or a low-humidity area of your fridge. Remove from plastic before storing.

BAKED POTATOES If you want to bake them in the oven, preheat the oven to 400°. Pierce the skin with a fork, then cover in foil or simply rub with olive oil. Place on a rimmed baking sheet and cook for about 60 minutes (sweet potatoes will be done sooner, in about 45 minutes). You'll know they're fully cooked when you pierce them with a knife and it slides out easily. For a truly delicious baked potato, try our Broccoli and Cheese–Stuffed Baked Potato recipe (page 188).

STOVETOP POTATOES You can also cook potatoes on the stovetop. Bring a large stockpot of generously salted water to a boil and place potatoes in one by one (red or new potatoes can go in whole, but cut or quarter larger potatoes). Simmer for 30 minutes or until potatoes can be pierced with a sharp knife.

MICROWAVE POTATOES Potatoes and sweet potatoes should be baked in the microwave on HIGH for about 10 minutes. Check small and medium potatoes at about the 5-minute mark to make sure they don't get overcooked.

Must-Have Tools for a *CarbLovers* Kitchen

The Essentials

BLENDER A blender is the best and easiest way to whip up the smoothies on page 66, and you don't need a fancy one to get most kitchen jobs done. Blenders are also great for creating homemade salad dressing or puréeing soups.

CAST-IRON SKILLET Low-maintenance, hard-working, and super-affordable, every cook needs a cast-iron skillet for searing, roasting, even baking (nothing is better for making real cornbread in the oven!). Bonus: These pans provide traces of iron, a nutrient many women don't get enough of.

DUTCH OVEN These large, heavy-bottomed pots belong in every kitchen. They go from stovetop to oven and last forever. Use them for everything from batch-cooking beans and oatmeal to searing meats and making roasts, casseroles, stews, and soups.

FOOD PROCESSOR Such a time-saver when you don't feel like chopping. If you don't want to get a large 16- to 20-cup processor, a mini 4-cup version will handle most of the recipes in this book.

FOOD-STORAGE CONTAINERS The ultimate time- and money-saver! A good selection will keep your leftovers or batch-cooked foods fresh, and allow you to carry *CarbLovers* meals to work or wherever you are headed. Be sure to choose containers that are BPA-free and have secure lids.

KNIVES Like most home cooks, *CarbLovers* cooks will do just fine with these three: a large chef's knife for slicing meat, fish, and vegetables; a paring knife for peeling and mincing smaller vegetables like garlic; and a serrated knife for slicing bread and pizza.

MUFFIN TIN Having at least one regular 12-cup tin is a must for baking up several weeks' worth of your favorite *CarbLovers* muffins, page 50.

Also great to have:

HERB CHOPPER Dried herbs are handy, but fresh will rock your world! These mini hand choppers make quick work of parsley, cilantro, basil, and other fresh herbs that add calorie- and sodium-free flavor to dishes.

IMMERSION BLENDER So much power for so little money! These handy wands, which often cost under $30, can purée an entire batch of soup or marinara sauce—right in the pot! If you use them to whip up smoothies, make sure to put the ingredients in an oversize glass or plastic container to avoid splashes.

SLOW COOKER There's a reason more than 80 percent of American households have one! Slow cookers are great for soups, stews, even casseroles. Just turn on in the morning, set on "low" or "high," and dinner is done when you get home from work. Try serving dinner straight from your cooker, family style!

PIZZA STONE Great for giving our Fresh Mozzarella, Basil, and Chicken Sausage Pizza (page 136) a crisp and chewy crust.

The Slim Way to Organize Your Kitchen

Your kitchen can be set up to make your *CarbLovers* cooking easy and even inspiring.

The first place to start? The refrigerator. First, ditch the soda—regular and diet (carbonation plus artificial sweeteners equals bloat), and replace it with water and iced green tea. Better yet, try the *CarbLovers* Fat-Flushing Cocktail: Take 2 quarts brewed green tea and add the juice of 1 lemon, 1 lime, and 1 orange. Mix all ingredients together in a large pitcher. Store in the fridge for up to 3 days. If you must keep soda and fruit juice around for your family, do yourself a favor and store them out of sight. That way, you'll be more likely to grab something diet-friendly.

Invest in fridge- and freezer-friendly stackable containers so the healthy stuff—chopped veggies, herbs, sliced fruit, and all your make-ahead beans, barley, and brown rice—is easier to grab than fattening fare. These will keep your fridge clutter-free, and encourage you to cook *CarbLovers* meals in large batches that you can use for the whole week. Look for the "make-ahead" icon on some of the recipes. These meals can be made in advance of serving, and many are appropriate for freezing.

Your next stop is the countertop: This is a space that can make or break your diet. Keep your blender close to where you chop fruits or veggies so it's always supereasy to prepare a healthy smoothie or soup. Set out a wooden block or hang a magnetic strip for chopping knives to make it easy to trim excess fat from meat and slice fiber-filled veggies and fruit.

Next to those slicers, use decorative hooks to dangle tools like an apple corer, a citrus zester, and a handheld squeezer (to add no-fat flavor to fish, pastas, marinades, and salad dressings).

Top your countertop with a big, beautiful basket, and use it to contain kitchen-table clutter, so you won't be tempted to multitask during meals. (Also recommended: a bouquet of fresh flowers, just because you deserve it.) Cooking and eating without distractions will help you focus! Speaking of focus, plug in your iPod and listen to music that de-stresses you. Research suggests that ab fat cells expand in response to the stress hormone cortisol, but cortisol levels decrease faster in people who listen to relaxing music than in those who don't.

> **TIP:**
> Grow your own oregano, thyme, and rosemary along your windowsill, and you'll have an easy, no-cal way to jazz up healthy foods like grilled chicken and veggies.

When it comes to the pantry, de-cluttering is key! Don't keep unhealthy snacks around to tempt you into mindless munching while you're cooking meals. Instead, keep airtight containers of dry ingredients like pasta and beans on the lowest shelves, so they're convenient for everyday use (check them periodically for freshness).

Build Your *CarbLovers* Kitchen

It's key to have a pantry and refrigerator stocked with the right foods. When healthy ingredients are at your fingertips, you won't be tempted to go off your diet. Make sure you have the following within reach at all times:

PANTRY

Almonds, walnuts, other nuts and seeds (unsalted)

Almond and peanut butter (natural)

Baked potato chips

Barley

Brown rice

Bulgur

Canned beans

Canned tomatoes

Coconut, shredded, unsweetened

Cornflakes

Dates

Dried beans

Dried herbs

Balsamic vinaigrette

Oatmeal (preferably rolled or steel-cut)

Olive oil, both regular and extra virgin

Polenta

Quinoa

Rye crispbread crackers

Tortilla chips, baked

Vinegar

Whole-grain bread

Whole-grain pasta

COUNTERTOP

Apples

Avocados

Bananas

Garlic

Onions

Pears

Potatoes and sweet potatoes

Tomatoes

REFRIGERATOR

Berries, fresh when in season. Use frozen when not.

Broccoli

Carrots

Celery

Fresh herbs

Lemons

Limes

Low-fat milk

Low-fat cheese

Olives

Salad greens

Salmon

Tortillas

Yogurt, preferably low-fat Greek

FREEZER

Batch-cooked beans and grains

Whole-grain pizza dough

Frozen fruit

Frozen veggies

Frozen *CarbLover*-approved meals (see page 314)

Recipe icons

Gluten-Free These recipes contain no wheat, spelt, kamut, farro, bulgur, semolina, barley, rye, or triticale. Some brands of other food products (such as oats, premade broths, canned beans, and condiments) may contain gluten, so if you have celiac disease, always buy products labeled gluten-free.

Kid-Friendly Designed to deter dinnertime melt-downs, our kid-friendly meals are yummy, uncomplicated, and healthy for the whole family.

Make-Ahead These meals can be made in advance, and many are appropriate for freezing.

Low-Sodium Defined as less than 500 mg for a meal or less than 250 mg per side or dessert.

Superfast Our collection of Superfast recipes take just 25 minutes (or less) total.

Vegetarian These recipes do not contain any meat or meat products (such as chicken broth), but they may include dairy and eggs. Look for tips on recipes for how to make some of our meat-based meals vegetarian.

PART 2
The *CarbLovers* Recipe Collection

Breakfast

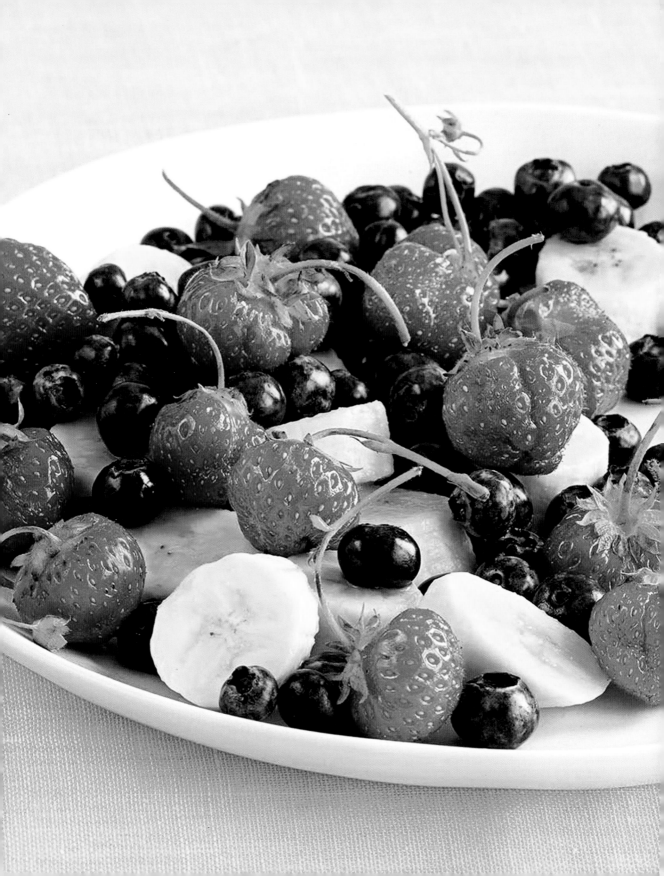

RS
7.6g

Oat and Honey Pancakes with Strawberry Syrup

Prep: 5 minutes | **Cook:** 15 minutes | **Total time:** 20 minutes | **Makes:** 6 servings

What could be better for breakfast than a stack of hot pancakes? A stack of pancakes packed with Resistant Starch! And this recipe also features a delicious (and simple) topping of antioxidant-rich strawberries.

Cooking spray
1   cup whole-wheat flour
½   cup all-purpose flour
¼   cup toasted wheat germ
2   cups old-fashioned rolled oats
1   tablespoon baking powder
½   teaspoon salt
½   teaspoon ground cinnamon
2   tablespoons honey
2   tablespoons sugar, divided
2   cups low-fat milk (1%)
2   large eggs
2   tablespoons vegetable oil
1   quart strawberries, hulled and
    quartered
1   tablespoon fresh lemon juice

1. Place flours, wheat germ, oats, baking powder, salt, and cinnamon in a food processor; process until combined. Whisk together honey, 1 tablespoon sugar, milk, eggs, and vegetable oil in a large bowl; stir in flour mixture until well combined. Let stand 5 minutes.

2. Meanwhile, combine strawberries, lemon juice, and remaining tablespoon sugar in a large bowl. Crush with clean hands; set aside.

3. Heat a nonstick griddle or skillet over medium heat. Coat pan with cooking spray. Pour about ¼ cup batter per pancake onto pan. Cook for 2 minutes or until tops are covered with bubbles and edges are cooked. Using a spatula, carefully turn pancakes over; cook 1 minute more or until bottoms are lightly browned. Transfer pancakes to a plate; keep warm. Repeat with remaining batter. Serve with strawberry topping (you will have some left over).

Serving size: About 3 pancakes, 4 tablespoons strawberry topping Calories: 395; Fat 10.6g (sat 2g, mono 2.9g, poly 4.7g); Cholesterol 66mg; Protein 14g; Carbohydrate 65g; Sugars 20g; Fiber 8g; RS 7.6g; Sodium 499mg

TIP:
Fresh strawberries are always best, but you can also use frozen, defrosted berries—they're just as nutritious.

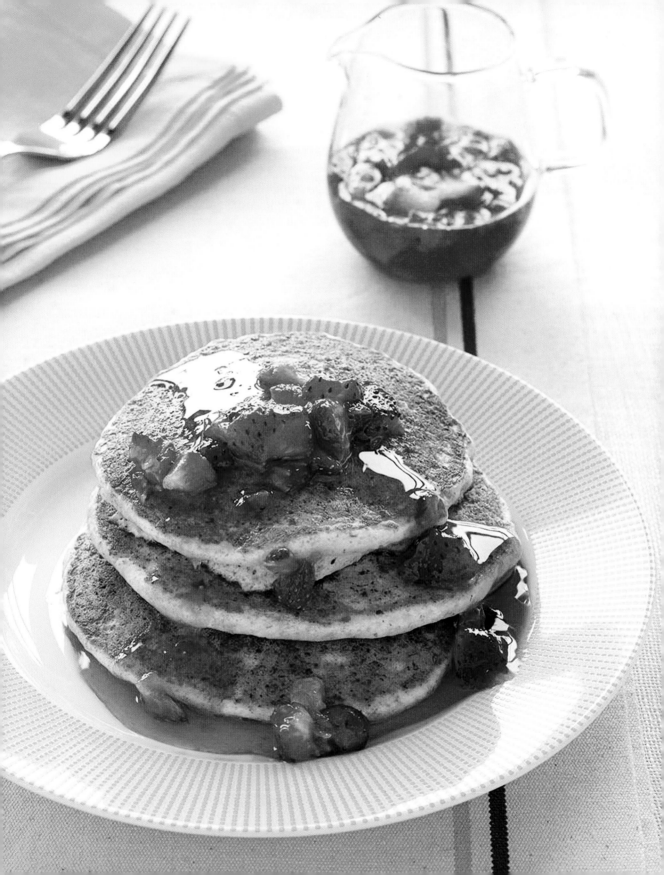

RS
0.6g

Eggs Benedict Florentine

Prep: 10 minutes | *Cook:* 10 minutes | *Total time:* 20 minutes | *Makes:* 4 servings

Eggs Benedict on a diet? Yes you can! We make ours with a light hollandaise that still tastes incredibly rich. This is the perfect dish for a special Sunday brunch.

1   teaspoon white vinegar
1   teaspoon olive oil
1   (5-ounce) container baby spinach
¼   teaspoon Kosher salt
⅛   teaspoon freshly ground black pepper
¼   teaspoon freshly grated nutmeg
4   slices sourdough bread, about 1 ounce each, toasted
5   large eggs
3   tablespoons light mayonnaise
1   tablespoon lemon juice
1   tablespoon melted butter

1. Bring a high-sided skillet filled with 2 inches of water to a simmer; add vinegar.

2. Heat oil in a large skillet over medium-high heat. Add spinach; season with salt and pepper. Cook, stirring, until spinach is wilted, about 3 minutes; stir in nutmeg. Arrange toasted bread on 4 plates; divide spinach among toast.

3. Break 1 egg into a ramekin and slide into simmering water. Gently poach 3 minutes; remove with a slotted spoon. Repeat with remaining eggs. Place 1 egg on each toasted slice; reserve last egg.

4. Combine yolk from remaining poached egg (discard white), mayonnaise, lemon juice, and 2 teaspoons water in a blender; blend until smooth. Add butter; blend to combine. Spoon hollandaise over eggs and serve immediately.

Serving size: 1 slice bread, ½ cup cooked spinach, 1 tablespoon hollandaise, 1 egg Calories 256; Fat 14.3g (sat 4.7g, mono 4.9g, poly 3.6g); Cholesterol 251mg; Protein 11g; Carbohydrate 21g; Sugars 2g; Fiber 2g; RS 0.6g; Sodium 471mg

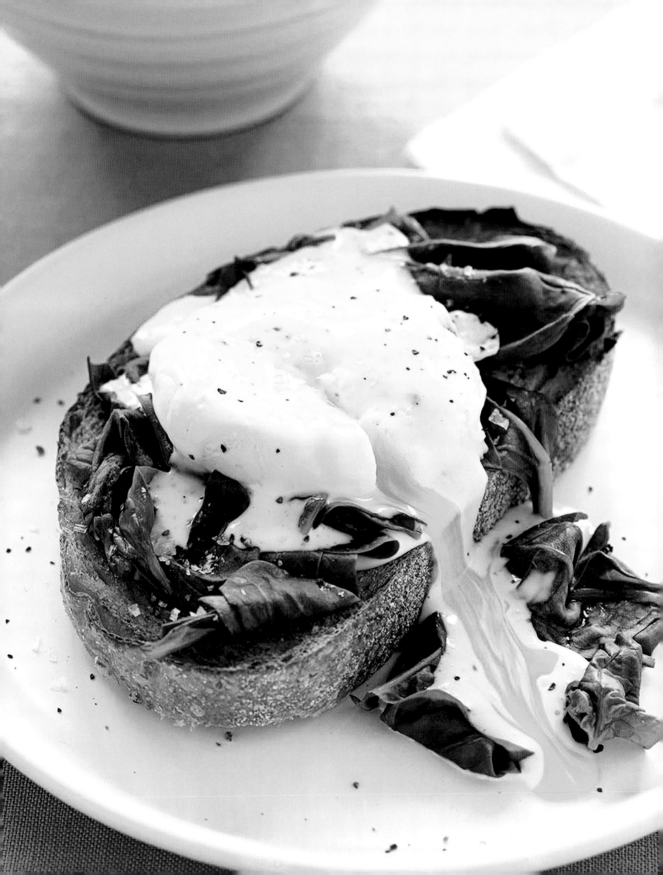

Steel-Cut Oatmeal with Salted Caramel Topping

Prep: 5 minutes | *Cook: 15 minutes* | *Total time: 20 minutes* | *Makes: 4 servings*

Decadent and healthy? They co-exist in this delicious breakfast. It's perfect for company, or just a quick midweek morning meal.

1 cup uncooked instant steel-cut oats
3 cups low-fat milk (1%)
¼ cup light brown sugar
½ teaspoon salt
¼ cup whipped cream
½ cup fresh berries

1. Preheat oven to 400°.

2. Combine oatmeal and milk in a medium saucepan. Bring to a boil over high heat. Reduce heat and simmer until oatmeal is cooked but not mushy, 7–8 minutes.

3. Remove from heat and distribute oatmeal among four 6-ounce ramekins. Arrange ramekins on a rimmed baking sheet.

4. Combine sugar and salt and sprinkle evenly on top of ramekins. Place ramekins (on baking sheet) in oven for 3–4 minutes, until sugar is melted.

5. Remove from oven and turn oven to broil. Return to oven and broil ramekins until sugar is browned and bubbly, watching carefully to keep them from burning, 2–3 minutes.

6. Remove from oven and top each oatmeal brûlée with 1 tablespoon whipped cream and 1 tablespoon berries. Serve warm.

Serving size: 1 ramekin Calories 242; Fat 5.9g (sat 3.1g, mono 1.7g, poly 0.7g); Cholesterol 19mg; Protein 9g; Carbohydrate 39g; Sugars 25g; Fiber 2g; RS 2.3g; Sodium 229mg

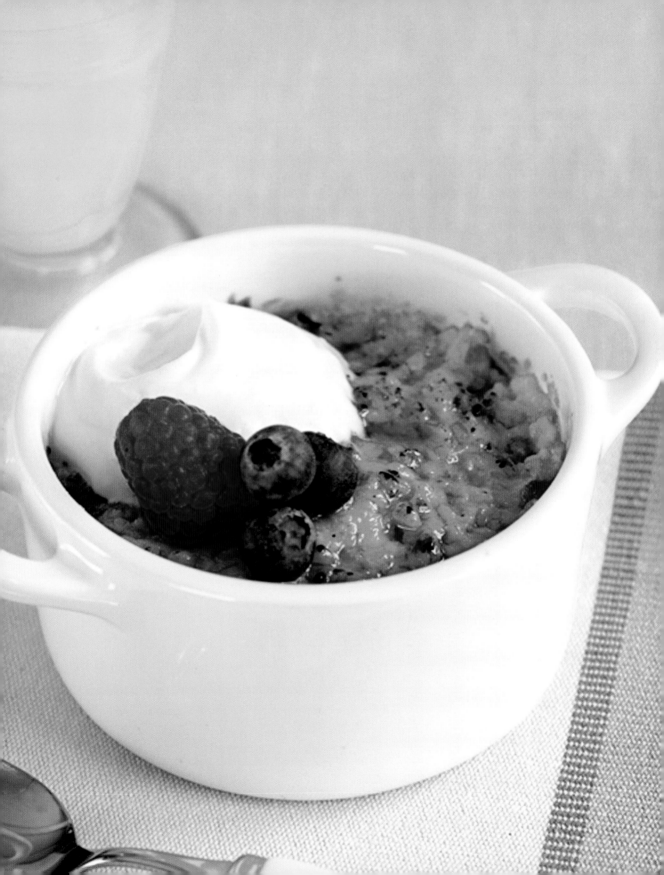

Fresh Citrus with Chopped Crystallized Ginger and Basil

Prep: *10 minutes* | **Total time:** *10 minutes* | **Makes:** *4 servings*

Sunny, bright, and packed with vitamin C, this simple fruit salad is a welcome dish at any brunch.

2 large grapefruits, segmented
2 large oranges, segmented
3 tablespoons (1 ounce) crystallized ginger, thinly sliced
1 tablespoon fresh basil ribbons

1. Gently combine grapefruit and orange segments in a medium bowl.

2. Divide fruit among 4 bowls. Sprinkle evenly with ginger and basil. Serve.

Serving size: About 1 cup Calories 111; Fat 0.3g (sat 0g, mono 0g, poly 0.1g); Cholesterol 0mg; Protein 2g; Carbohydrate 28g; Sugars 20g; Fiber 3g; RS 0g; Sodium 3mg

ASK CARBLOVERS

Q: How much fruit can I eat on *CarbLovers*?

A: Our daily plans include 5–6 servings of fruit and vegetables. Fruit is rich in antioxidants and high in fiber, which will help you stay full. It's not unlimited on the diet, but you can eat three servings each day. A medium-size piece of fruit or ½ cup of sliced fruit equals a serving.

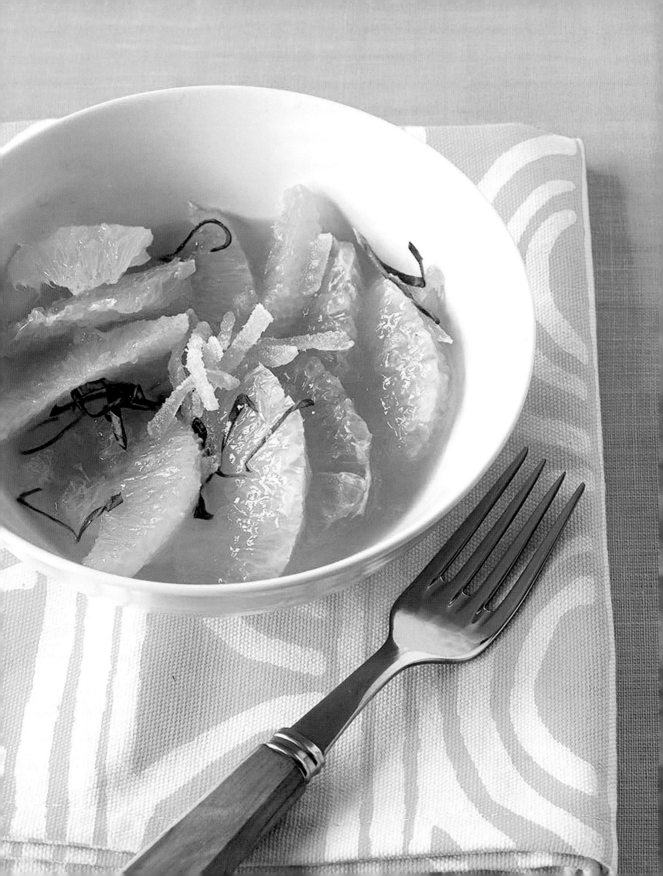

RS
2.7g

Huevos Rancheros

Prep: 10 minutes | *Cook:* 15 minutes | *Total time:* 25 minutes | *Makes:* 4 servings

Love this Mexican classic? While our version is hearty and filling (and fiber- and protein-packed), we've lightened it up by toasting—not frying—the tortillas and using cooking spray instead of oil for the eggs.

2	teaspoons vegetable oil
½	cup finely diced onion
2	garlic cloves, minced
¼	teaspoon cumin
¼	teaspoon chipotle chile powder
⅛	teaspoon salt
1	(15-ounce) can low-sodium black beans, rinsed and drained
½	cup low-sodium chicken broth
1	tablespoon chopped cilantro, plus more for garnish
	Cooking spray
8	eggs
8	corn tortillas, warmed in pan
1	cup jarred tomatillo salsa
1	cup chopped tomato
1	medium avocado, sliced

1. Heat oil in a small saucepan over medium-high heat. Add onion and cook, stirring, until softened, 6–7 minutes. Add garlic, cumin, chipotle chile powder, and salt; cook 1 more minute. Add beans and broth and bring to a boil. Reduce heat and cook until most of liquid is absorbed, 3–4 minutes. Remove from heat, add cilantro, and reserve.

2. Heat a large nonstick skillet coated with cooking spray over medium-high heat. Crack 2 eggs in pan; cook as desired, either sunny-side up or over easy. Repeat with remaining eggs.

3. For each serving: Arrange 2 warmed tortillas on a large plate and slide 1 egg onto each tortilla. To each plate, add ⅓ cup bean mixture, ¼ cup salsa, ¼ cup tomato, and ¼ of the avocado. Garnish with additional cilantro and serve.

Serving size: 2 tortillas, 2 eggs, ⅓ cup bean mixture, and toppings Calories 467; Fat 20g (sat 4.3g, mono 8.2g, poly 4.7g); Cholesterol 372mg; Protein 22g; Carbohydrate 50g; Sugars 7g; Fiber 11g; RS 2.7g; Sodium 710mg

> **TIP:**
> This is a big breakfast, so if you're on the Kickstart, or just want to go lighter, split it with a friend.

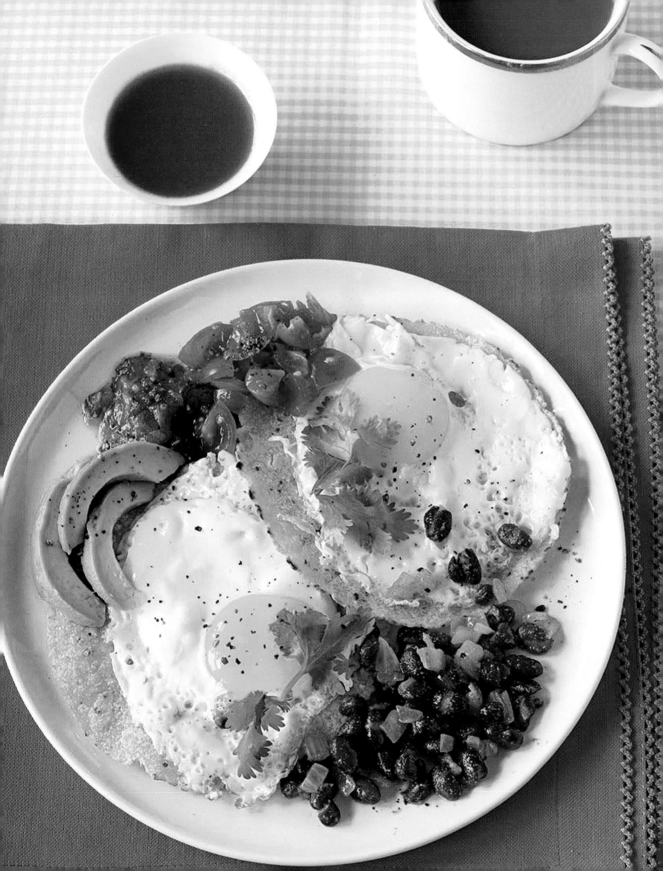

RS
4.6g

Granola with Pecans, Pumpkin Seeds, and Dried Mango

Prep: 5 minutes | **Cook:** 25 minutes | **Total time:** 30 minutes | **Makes:** 6 servings (3 cups total)

Crunchy nuts and chewy mango give a flavor-packed start to your day. This granola also makes a great snack; just cut the portion size to ¼ cup.

3 cups old-fashioned rolled oats
3 cups puffed millet cereal
⅓ cup lightly toasted chopped pecans
2 tablespoons pumpkin seeds
1 tablespoon canola oil
5 tablespoons pure maple syrup
3 tablespoons apple juice or apple cider
1 teaspoon pure vanilla extract
¼ teaspoon salt
3 tablespoons chopped dried mango

1. Preheat oven to 350°.

2. Line a large rimmed baking sheet with parchment paper and reserve.

3. Combine oats, cereal, pecans, and pumpkin seeds in a large bowl.

4. Whisk together oil, syrup, juice, vanilla, and salt in a small bowl; toss with dry ingredients.

5. Spread on the prepared baking sheet and bake until golden brown, stirring occasionally, 20–25 minutes.

6. Remove from oven, let cool completely, and toss with mango.

Serving size: ½ cup granola Calories 330; Fat 11g (sat 1.3g, mono 5.3g, poly 3.7g); Cholesterol 0mg; Protein 8g; Carbohydrate 52g; Sugars 14g; Fiber 5g; RS 4.6g; Sodium 54mg

TIP:
This delicious granola can be stored in an airtight container for up to a week.

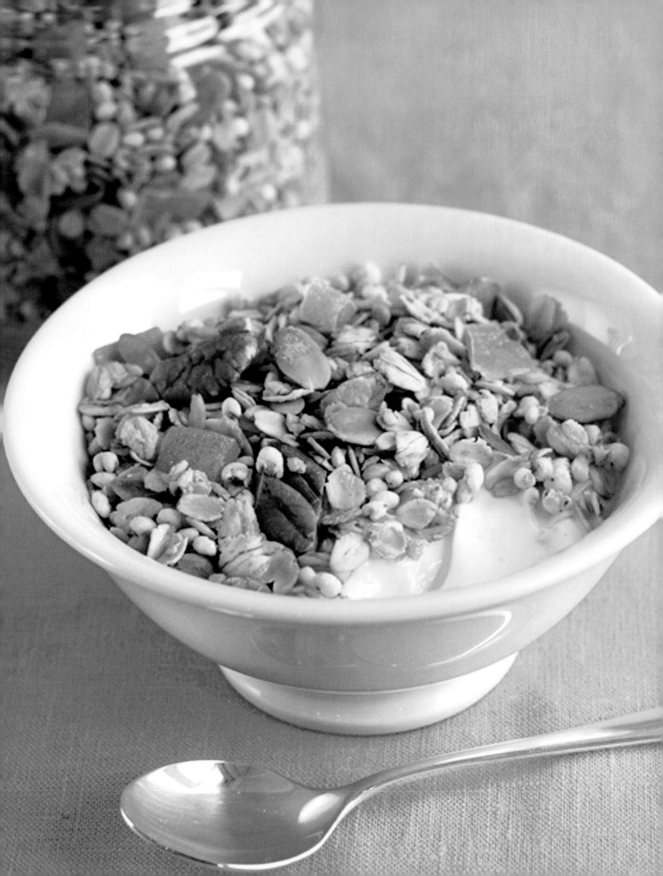

RS
0.2g

Asparagus, Mushroom, and Tomato Frittata

Prep: *10 minutes* | **Cook:** *30 minutes* | **Total time:** *40 minutes* | **Makes:** *6 servings*

If you want a big, hearty breakfast that also looks gorgeous on the table, a frittata is the way to go. Plus, it cooks up really quickly.

6 eggs

6 egg whites

1 ounce Parmesan cheese, finely shredded (about ½ cup)

½ teaspoon freshly ground black pepper

½ cup sliced basil leaves

2 tablespoons olive oil, divided

1 small onion, diced

6 slices (3 ounces) turkey bacon, diced

2 cups sliced mushrooms

1 cup (4 ounces) cooked, sliced potato

½ pound asparagus, trimmed and cut into 1½-inch pieces

1 cup small cherry or grape tomatoes

1. Preheat oven to 400°. Whisk together eggs, egg whites, cheese, pepper, and basil; reserve in refrigerator until ready to use.

2. Heat 1 tablespoon oil in a 10-inch cast-iron skillet or oven-safe pan over medium-high heat. Add onion and cook, stirring, until soft and slightly golden, 7–9 minutes.

3. Add turkey bacon and cook, stirring, until crisped, 4–5 minutes. Add mushrooms and cook until softened, 3–4 minutes. Add potato, asparagus, and tomatoes; cook 2 more minutes until asparagus just begins to soften.

4. Add remaining oil to skillet and stir to incorporate with bacon and vegetables. Add egg mixture and tilt pan to evenly distribute eggs. Cook until eggs just begin to set, 3–4 minutes. Transfer to oven and bake until top is lightly browned and eggs are fully set, 11–12 minutes.

5. Remove from oven and let cool slightly. Cut into 6 equal-size wedges. (Note: Can be served warm or at room temperature.)

Serving size: 1 wedge Calories 220; Fat 13.7g (sat 3.8g, mono 6.6g, poly 2.2g); Cholesterol 202mg; Protein 16g; Carbohydrate 9g; Sugars 3g; Fiber 2g; RS 0.2g; Sodium 384 mg

TIP:
This is a brilliant make-ahead dish for dinner or brunch. Prepare the day before, cover tightly with foil, refrigerate, then reheat in a 400° oven for 11–12 minutes.

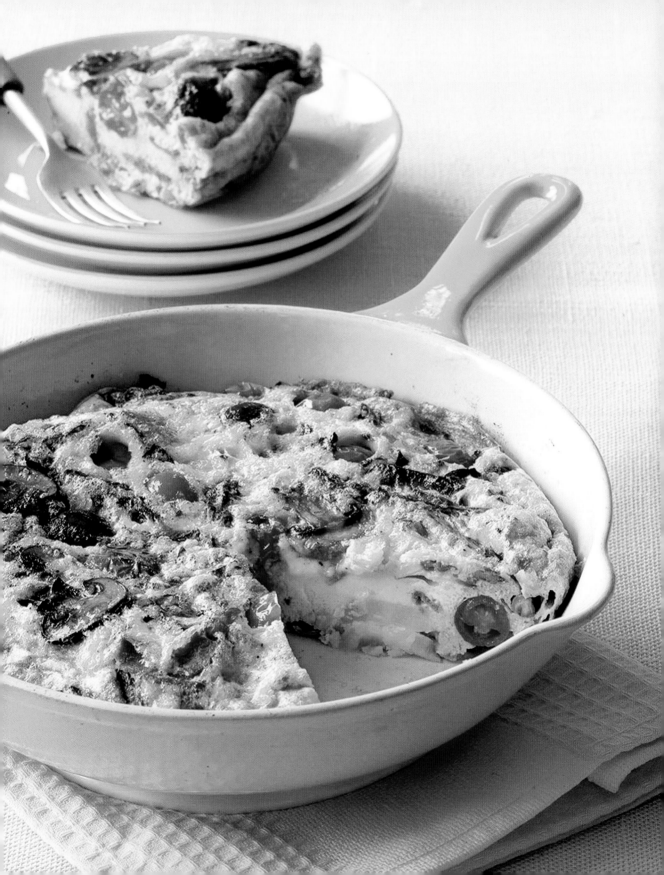

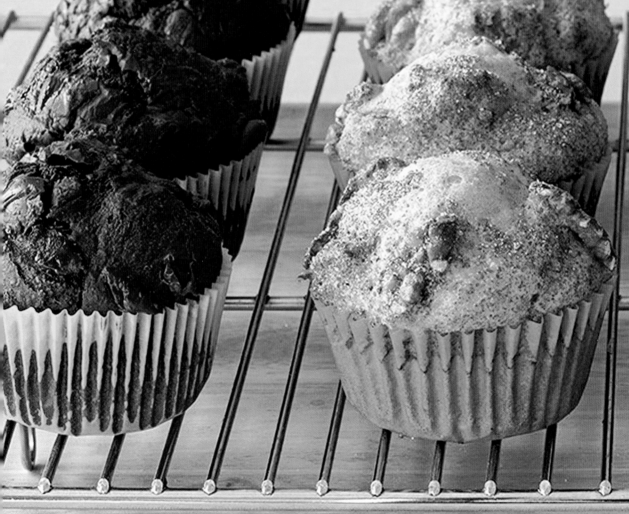

Double Chocolate Cherry

Cinnamon-Apple Walnut

Apricot-Pistachio

Blueberry

CarbLovers Muffin Collection!

Prep: 5 minutes | *Cook:* 16–20 minutes | *Total Time:* 25 minutes + 5 to cool | *Makes:* 12 muffins

Everyone needs a go-to muffin recipe for special mornings. Start with one great basic recipe and add extras for four delicious variations. Try them all!

Base

- ¾ cup all-purpose flour
- ½ cup white whole-wheat flour
- ½ cup sugar
- 1¼ teaspoons baking powder
- ¼ teaspoon ground nutmeg
- ½ teaspoon salt
- 1 large egg, lightly beaten
- ¾ cup soy milk
- 2 tablespoons vegetable oil
- 1 teaspoon pure vanilla extract

MIX-INS: STIR IN THESE INGREDIENTS WHEN YOU GET TO STEP 3 (RIGHT).

Double Chocolate Cherry

*Reduce all-purpose flour in base to ½ cup
- ½ cup semisweet chocolate chips
- ½ cup dried cherries
- ¼ cup unsweetened cocoa (add to flour mixture)

Serving size: 1 muffin Calories 165; Fat 5.4g (sat 1.6g, mono 1.4g, poly 1.8g); Cholesterol 16mg; Protein 3g; Carbohydrate 27g; Sugars 16g; Fiber 2g; RS 0g; Sodium 173mg

Cinnamon- Apple Walnut

- ½ cup chopped dried apples
- ½ cup chopped walnuts
- 1 tablespoon sugar + ½ teaspoon cinnamon for topping

Serving size: 1 muffin Calories 159; Fat 6.3g (sat 0.6g, mono 1.2g, poly 4g); Cholesterol 16mg; Protein 3g; Carbohydrate 24g; Sugars 12g; Fiber 2g; RS 0g; Sodium 175mg

Apricot-Pistachio

- ½ cup chopped dried apricots
- ½ cup chopped pistachios
- 2 tablespoons shredded unsweetened coconut for topping

Serving size: 1 muffin Calories 162; Fat 6g (sat 1.1g, mono 2g, poly 2.4g); Cholesterol 16mg; Protein 4g; Carbohydrate 24g; Sugars 13g; Fiber 2g; RS 0g; Sodium 172mg

Blueberry

- 1 cup fresh blueberries

Serving size: 1 muffin Calories 121; Fat 3.2g (sat 0.4g, mono 0.7g, poly 1.8g); Cholesterol 16mg; Protein 3g; Carbohydrate 21g; Sugars 10g; Fiber 1g; RS 0g; Sodium 172mg

1. Preheat oven to 400°. Line a 12-cup muffin pan with paper liners.

2. Combine flours and next 4 ingredients (through salt) in a large bowl; stir with a whisk. Make a well in center of mixture.

3. Add egg, milk, oil, and vanilla to flour mixture, stirring until just combined. Stir in mix-in ingredients. Divide batter evenly among prepared muffin pan. Add topping as indicated.

4. Bake 16–20 minutes or until a wooden pick inserted in the center of a muffin comes out clean. Cool in pans on a wire rack for 5 minutes; remove muffins from pans and cool completely on rack.

Juicy berries add flavor
and antioxidants
to this healthy and
yummy muffin.

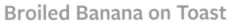

RS
4g

Broiled Banana on Toast

Prep: 5 minutes | **Cook:** 5 minutes | **Total time:** 10 minutes | **Makes:** 1 serving

No time for breakfast? Try this superfast and yummy open-faced sandwich, which is packed with Resistant Starch from both the bananas and the rye bread.

1   tablespoon brown sugar
½   large banana, removed
     from peel and halved lengthwise
1   slice rye bread (1.5 ounces),
     toasted
2   tablespoons reduced-fat
     peanut butter

1. Preheat broiler with rack 4 inches from heat source. Place sugar on a plate; dip cut sides of bananas in sugar. Arrange banana cut side up on a baking sheet or in a broiler-proof baking dish; broil 3–5 minutes, rotating sheet often, until banana is browned.

2. Spread toast with peanut butter; top with banana.

Serving size: 1 slice toast Calories 413; Fat 13.6g (sat 2.3g, mono 6.6g, poly 3.9g); Cholesterol 0mg; Protein 12g; Carbohydrate 62g; Sugars 25g; Fiber 6g; RS 4g; Sodium 400mg

ASK CARBLOVERS

Q: **I'm not a fan of bananas. What can I do?**

A: Bananas are an incredible source of Resistant Starch, but if you don't love 'em, no worries. In this recipe, you could easily substitute an apple or a pear for the banana. Just make sure you're getting enough RS each day from other sources.

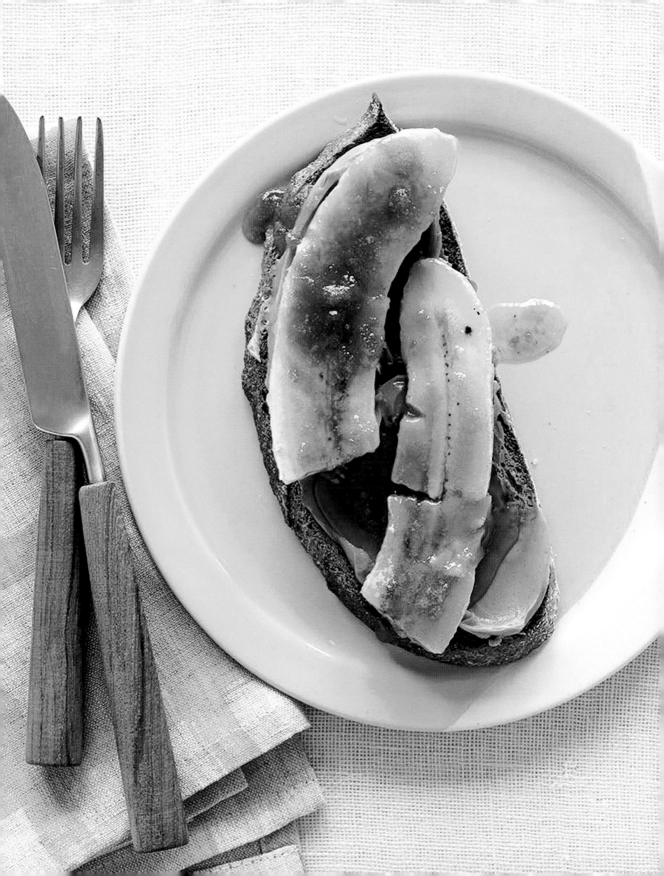

RS
0.3g

Toad in the Hole

Prep: *5 minutes* | **Cook:** *15 minutes* | **Total time:** *20 minutes* | **Makes:** *4 servings*

The name is a total hoot, but trust us, this classic breakfast is the ultimate comfort meal.

Cooking spray
8 large cherry tomatoes, halved
4 slices whole-grain bread
4 teaspoons melted butter
4 eggs

1. Coat a large nonstick pan with cooking spray. Heat pan to medium-high heat; add tomatoes. Cook until just soft and hot, 3–5 minutes. Remove from pan and keep warm.

2. Using a 2-inch cookie cutter, carefully cut circles from each slice of bread. Brush bread and cutouts with butter and place facedown in pan. Toast until golden, 2–3 minutes. Flip bread slices and crack an egg into the center (the "hole") of each piece. Cook until eggs are partially done, 2–3 minutes. Using a spatula, carefully flip egg-filled toasts and cutouts. Continue cooking until whites are cooked through, 1–2 more minutes. Sprinkle with salt and pepper, if desired.

3. Remove from pan and place each toast on a plate, along with a cutout. Serve with tomatoes.

Serving size: 1 slice bread and egg, plus cutout and 2 tomatoes Calories 184; Fat 10.1g (sat 4.2g, mono 3g, poly 1.6g); Cholesterol 196mg; Protein 10g; Carbohydrate 13g; Sugars 3g; Fiber 2g; RS 0.3g; Sodium 182mg

ASK CARBLOVERS

Q: **Can I eat breakfast for dinner—and vice versa—on *CarbLovers*?**

A: Sure! Some people feel more in control when they eat the same thing every day—even if it's a shake for dinner or pasta for breakfast! If that sounds like you, then go for it. It will almost certainly make it easier for you to stick to the plan.

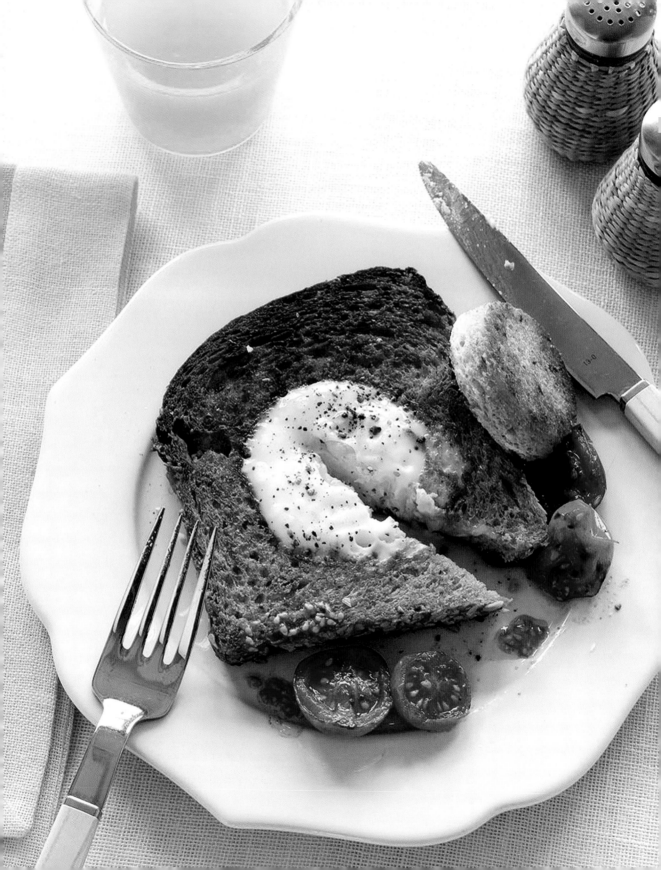

RS
1.2g

Tartine with Blackberry Thyme Salad

Prep: 3 minutes | Total time: 3 minutes | Makes: 4 servings

Celebrate berry season with this delicious no-cook breakfast sandwich. You can substitute blueberries if you can't find blackberries.

1 quart fresh blackberries
1 tablespoon fresh thyme leaves
2 teaspoons sugar
1 tablespoon fresh lemon juice
   Pinch of kosher salt
1 sourdough baguette (about 8 ounces), split lengthwise and cut into 4 pieces
2 tablespoons softened butter
24 ounces plain low-fat yogurt

1. With clean hands or a spatula, crush blackberries, thyme, sugar, lemon juice, and salt together in a medium bowl. Spread each baguette piece with ½ tablespoon butter and top with ¼ of the blackberry salad. Serve with ¼ of the yogurt.

Serving size: 1 tartine and 6 ounces plain low-fat yogurt
Calories 393; Fat 10.2g (sat 5.6g, mono 2.5g, poly 1.1g); Cholesterol 25mg; Protein 18g; Carbohydrate 60g; Sugars 22g; Fiber 9g; RS 1.2g; Sodium 418mg

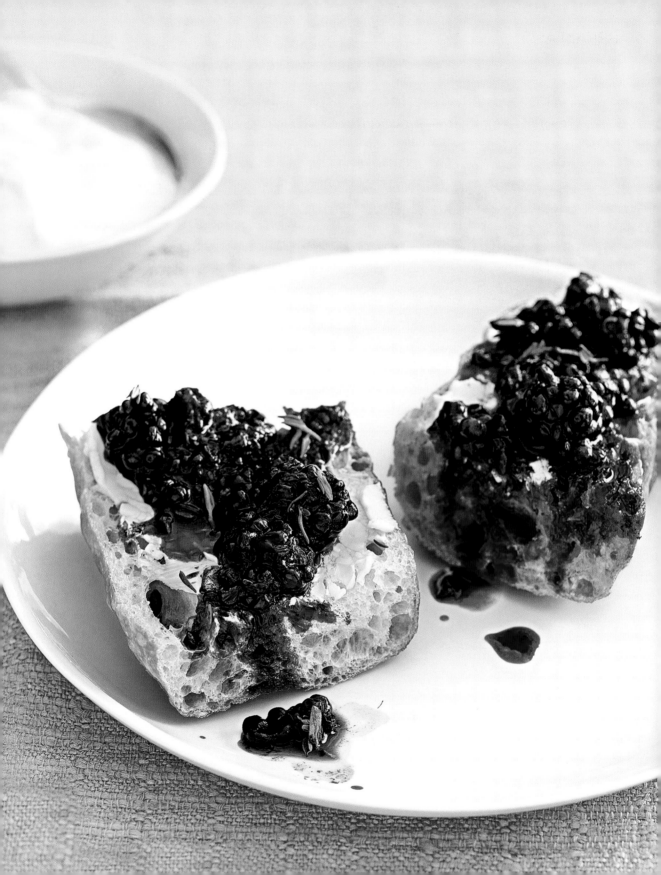

Whole-Grain Waffles with Caramelized Pineapple

Prep: 10 minutes | *Cook:* 20 minutes | *Total time:* 30 minutes | *Makes:* 8 servings

Want a special CarbLovers *weekend brunch? Try these delicious waffles.*

FOR TOPPING:

- 2 tablespoons melted butter
- 3 tablespoons dark brown sugar
- ½ teaspoon pure vanilla extract
- 8 ounces pineapple chunks (about 1 cup), fresh or frozen, thawed

FOR WAFFLES:

- ¾ cup all-purpose flour
- ¾ cup whole-wheat flour
- 2 tablespoons wheat germ
- 1½ teaspoons baking powder
- ½ teaspoon baking soda
- ¼ teaspoon salt
- 2 cups buttermilk, plus more for loosening batter if necessary
- 2 tablespoons melted butter
- 1 tablespoon pure maple syrup
- 2 egg whites
- 1 teaspoon pure vanilla extract
  Cooking spray

MAKE TOPPING:

1. Combine butter, brown sugar, and vanilla in a saucepan and bring to a boil. Reduce heat, add pineapple to coat, and cook until pineapple is golden brown, 3–4 minutes.

MAKE WAFFLES:

1. Preheat a waffle iron.

2. Place flours, wheat germ, baking powder, baking soda, and salt in a bowl; whisk to combine. Place buttermilk, butter, maple syrup, egg whites, and vanilla in a separate bowl; whisk to combine. Combine dry and wet ingredients; whisk until just incorporated (batter will be thick).

3. Coat waffle iron with cooking spray; pour ¼ of the batter into waffle iron. Cook until golden brown, about 3–4 minutes. Transfer to a plate and keep warm. Repeat with remaining batter.

4. Stack two waffle quarters (or squares) on top of each other. Drizzle with ¼ cup pineapple topping and serve.

Serving size: 2 waffle quarters with ¼ cup pineapple topping Calories 216; Fat 7.3g (sat 4.1g, mono 2g, poly 0.6g); Cholesterol 18mg; Protein 6g; Carbohydrate 32g; Sugars 13g; Fiber 2g; RS 0g; Sodium 336mg

> **TIP:**
> You can substitute other fruit for the pineapple. Bananas, blueberries, and apples are all amazing with these waffles.

Banana-Pecan Breakfast Bread

RS
0.9g

***Prep:** 10 minutes* | ***Cook:** 60 minutes* | ***Total Time:** 70 minutes + time to cool* | ***Makes:** 16 servings*

Fresh, warm banana bread is a special way to start your day. And it makes great use of your too-ripe bananas!

1	cup all-purpose flour
½	cup white whole-wheat flour
½	cup wheat germ
½	cup sugar
½	teaspoon salt
½	teaspoon baking powder
¼	teaspoon baking soda
1½	cups mashed ripe bananas (from 3-4 medium bananas)
⅓	cup vegetable oil
2	large eggs, lightly beaten
⅓	cup coarsely chopped pecans
	Cooking spray

1. Preheat oven to 350°.

2. Combine flours, wheat germ, sugar, salt, baking powder, and baking soda in a large bowl; make a well in center of mixture. Combine bananas, oil, and eggs in a separate bowl; add to flour mixture. Stir until just moist, then stir in pecans.

3. Coat an 8- by 4-inch loaf pan with cooking spray; spoon in batter. Bake at 350° for 1 hour or until a wooden pick inserted in center comes out clean. Cool bread in pan 10 minutes on a wire rack. Remove bread from pan; cool completely on rack.

Serving size: 1 slice Calories 168; Fat 7.5g (sat 0.8g, mono 2.4g, poly 3.8g); Cholesterol 23mg; Protein 3g; Carbohydrate 23g; Sugars 9g; Fiber 2g; RS 0.9g; Sodium 119mg

TIP:
Make two loaves at a time: Cool the second one, wrap in plastic wrap, then freeze. Bring to room temperature before serving.

RS
0.6g

Spinach and Egg Breakfast Wrap with Avocado and Pepper Jack Cheese

Prep: *10 minutes* | **Cook:** *5 minutes* | **Total time:** *15 minutes* | **Makes:** *4 servings*

We love breakfast sandwiches, so we created this fast take on a burrito, layering it with spicy cheese and creamy avocado. Serve with salsa for an extra kick.

Cooking spray
1 (5-ounce) container or bag baby spinach, chopped
4 eggs
4 egg whites
½ teaspoon salt
¼ teaspoon freshly ground black pepper
4 whole-wheat tortillas
4 ounces shredded pepper jack cheese
1 avocado, sliced
Hot sauce or salsa (optional)

1. Heat a nonstick skillet coated with cooking spray over medium-high heat.

2. Add spinach and cook, stirring, until wilted, 2 minutes.

3. Whisk together eggs and egg whites in a small bowl. Add eggs to skillet and cook, stirring, until cooked through, 3–4 minutes. Season with salt and pepper.

4. Place ¼ of egg mixture in the center of each tortilla; sprinkle with 1 ounce cheese.

5. Top each tortilla with 4 slices avocado and fold, burrito-style. Slice in half and serve.

Serving size: 1 wrap Calories 366; Fat 21.8g (sat 7.7g, mono 6.9g, poly 1.8g); Cholesterol 242mg; Protein 22g; Carbohydrate 30g; Sugars 1g; Fiber 7g; RS 0.6g; Sodium 666mg

TIP:
If you don't like spicy cheese, swap cheddar or Monterey Jack for pepper jack.

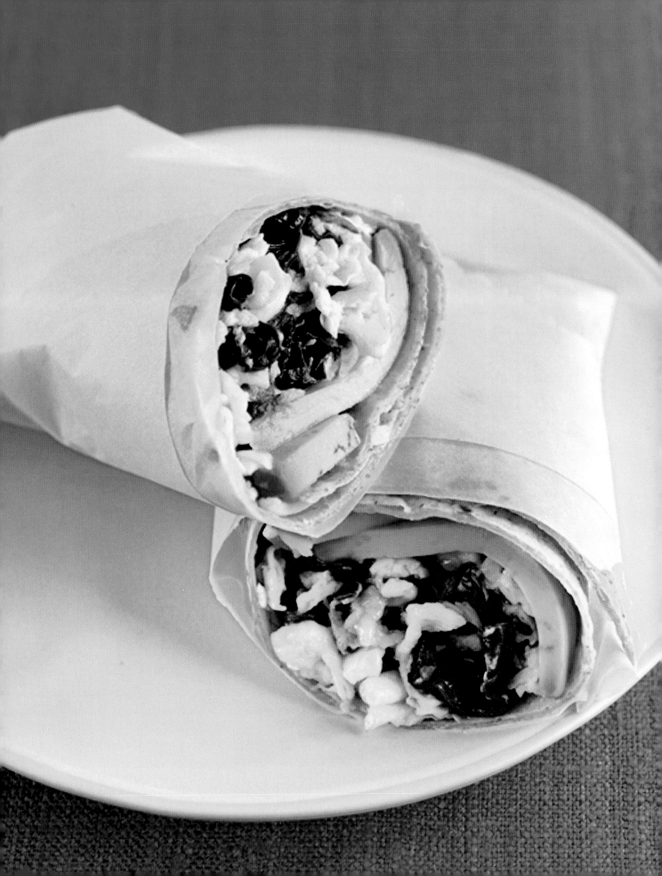

Buckwheat Crepes with Orange-Ricotta Filling

Prep: *10 minutes* | **Cook:** *10 minutes* | **Total time:** *20 minutes* | **Makes:** *6 servings*

Crepes might sound cooking-school complicated, but they're just as easy to make as pancakes.

- 2 cups part-skim ricotta
- 2 teaspoons finely grated orange zest
- 2 tablespoons fresh-squeezed orange juice
- 2 tablespoons powdered sugar, plus more for dusting
- ½ cup buckwheat flour
- ½ cup all-purpose flour
- 2 large eggs
- 3 tablespoons vegetable oil
- 1 cup fat-free milk
- ½ teaspoon salt
  Cooking spray
- 1 cup orange segments (from 2 oranges)

1. Make filling: Stir together ricotta, orange zest, orange juice, and sugar in a medium bowl. Cover and refrigerate mixture until ready to serve.

2. Make batter: Whisk together flours, eggs, oil, milk, 2 tablespoons water, and salt in a large bowl until well combined. Let stand 5 minutes.

3. Heat a 10-inch nonstick skillet over medium-high heat; coat pan with cooking spray. Pour about ⅓ cup batter per crepe onto pan. Cook 30–45 seconds or until crepe is golden on the bottom. Carefully turn crepe over with a spatula; cook 30 seconds or until bottom is lightly browned. Transfer crepes to a plate; keep warm. Repeat with remaining batter.

4. To assemble, spoon about ⅓ cup filling down the center of each crepe; roll up to form a cylinder. Place each rolled crepe on a plate, top with a few orange segments, dust with powdered sugar, and serve.

Serving size: 1 crepe and ⅓ cup filling, 3–5 orange segments Calories 322; Fat 15.7g (sat 5.2g, mono 4.4g, poly 5.2g); Cholesterol 88mg; Protein 16g; Carbohydrate 31g; Sugars 9g; Fiber 2g; RS 0g; Sodium 340mg

TIP:
With a sharp knife, segment your orange by slicing off the top and bottom, trimming away the peel and white pith, and releasing the pretty segments from the membrane.

Oatmeal-Cranberry Muffins

Prep: *5 minutes* | **Cook:** *30 minutes* | **Total time:** *35 minutes* | **Makes:** *12 muffins*

Make a batch of these on Sunday, and you'll have a healthy grab-and-go breakfast all week. Spread a tablespoon of almond or peanut butter on top for extra protein.

Cooking spray
1½ cups old-fashioned rolled oats
¾ cup all-purpose flour
¾ cup whole wheat flour
⅓ cup sugar
2½ teaspoons baking powder
1 teaspoon ground cinnamon
½ teaspoon ground nutmeg
½ teaspoon salt
½ cup oil
½ cup applesauce
2 eggs
½ cup dried, sweetened cranberries

1. Preheat oven to 350°.

2. Coat a 12-cup muffin pan with cooking spray and set aside.

3. Combine oats, flours, sugar, baking powder, spices, and salt in a bowl.

4. Whisk 1 cup water, oil, applesauce, and eggs in a separate bowl until incorporated.

5. Combine wet and dry ingredients; add cranberries.

6. Distribute batter evenly among muffin cups. Bake until a toothpick inserted in the center of a muffin comes out clean and tops are browned, 30–35 minutes.

Serving size: 1 muffin Calories 227; Fat 11.2g (sat 1.4g, mono 4.6g, poly 4.5g); Cholesterol 35mg; Protein 4g; Carbohydrate 29g; Sugars 10g; Fiber 3g; RS 1.2g; Sodium 194mg

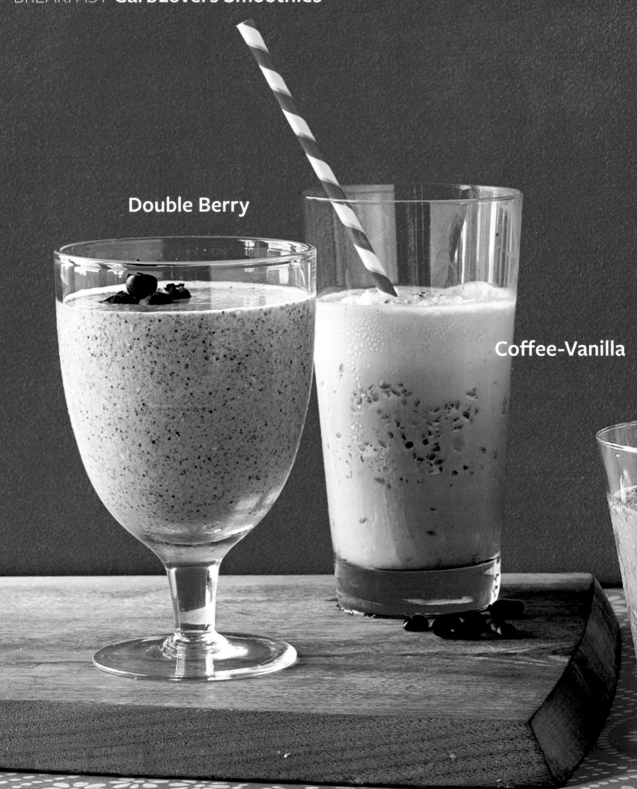

BREAKFAST **CarbLovers Smoothies**

Double Berry

Coffee-Vanilla

Peanut Butter–Banana Blast

Tropical Breeze

Chocolate
Antioxidant
Boost

CarbLovers Smoothies 5 Exciting Ways

Prep: 5 minutes | **Total time:** 5 minutes | **Makes:** 1 serving

Wake up to something wonderful! These five energizing smoothie combos will get you fueled up for whatever your day has in store.

Base

- 1 cup plain low-fat yogurt
- 1 teaspoon honey
- 1 teaspoon pure vanilla extract

Combine base ingredients and add-in ingredients in a blender; blend until smooth. Serve immediately.

MIX-INS:

Double Berry

- ¼ cup prepared quick-cooking oats, cooled
- 1 additional tablespoon honey
- ½ cup frozen blueberries
- ½ cup frozen strawberries
- ¼ cup skim milk

Serving size: About 16 ounces
Calories 371; Fat 5.2g (sat 2.7g, mono 1.3g, poly 0.4g); Cholesterol 16mg; Protein 18g; Carbohydrate 66g; Sugars 53g; Fiber 5g; RS 0.1g; Sodium 201mg

Coffee-Vanilla
(This one's for caffeine-loving adults only!)

- 3 tablespoons vanilla whey protein powder
- 1 tablespoon ground flax seed
- ¾ teaspoon espresso powder
- ½ cup ice

Serving size: About 16 ounces
Calories 299; Fat 8.1g (sat 3.4g, mono 1.7g, poly 2.4g); Cholesterol 36mg; Protein 25g; Carbohydrate 30g; Sugars 26g; Fiber 2g; RS 0g; Sodium 199mg

Chocolate Antioxidant Boost

- 2 teaspoons natural unsweetened cocoa
- 5 teaspoons additional honey
- 1 frozen unsweetened açaí smoothie pack (such as Sambazon)
- ⅓ cup ice

Serving size: About 16 ounces
Calories 382; Fat 10.1g (sat 4g, mono 4.5g, poly 1g); Cholesterol 15mg; Protein 15g; Carbohydrate 58g; Sugars 54g; Fiber 2g; RS 0g; Sodium 184mg

Peanut Butter–Banana Blast

- 1 cup sliced frozen bananas
- 2 tablespoons peanut butter
- ¼ cup ice

Serving size: About 16 ounces
Calories 509; Fat 20.4g (sat 6g, mono 8.8g, poly 4.8g); Cholesterol 15mg; Protein 23g; Carbohydrate 64g; Sugars 45g; Fiber 6g; RS 6g; Sodium 321mg

Tropical Breeze

- ½ cup pineapple chunks
- ½ cup mango chunks
- ¼ cup ice

Serving size: About 16 ounces
Calories 278; Fat 4.2g (sat 2.5g, mono 1.2g, poly 0.2g); Cholesterol 15mg; Protein 14g; Carbohydrate 47g; Sugars 43g; Fiber 2g; RS 0g; Sodium 174mg

On the run? Blend your smoothie, transfer to a tall lidded container, and go! Shake before drinking.

RS
1.2g

Berry-Kale Smoothie

Prep: 5 minutes | Total time: 5 minutes | Makes: 2 servings

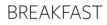

If you're looking for a quick, high-fiber breakfast, get out your blender and whip up this tasty shake. And please don't be afraid of the kale—you'll never know it's in there!

1½ cups fresh or frozen raspberries
½ cup shredded kale
1 cup ice
¾ cup fat-free plain yogurt
½ banana
2 tablespoons honey
1 tablespoon natural almond butter
1 tablespoon wheat germ

Combine all ingredients in a blender; blend until smooth. Serve immediately.

Serving size: 8 ounces Calories 248; Fat 5.6g (sat 0.5g, mono 2.7g, poly 1.8g); Cholesterol 2mg; Protein 9g; Carbohydrate 47g; Sugars 30g; Fiber 8g; RS 1.2g; Sodium 77mg

> **TIP:**
> This smoothie is also great for a lovely, light lunch, but for a complete meal, we suggest adding a whole-wheat English muffin with 1 tablespoon hummus.

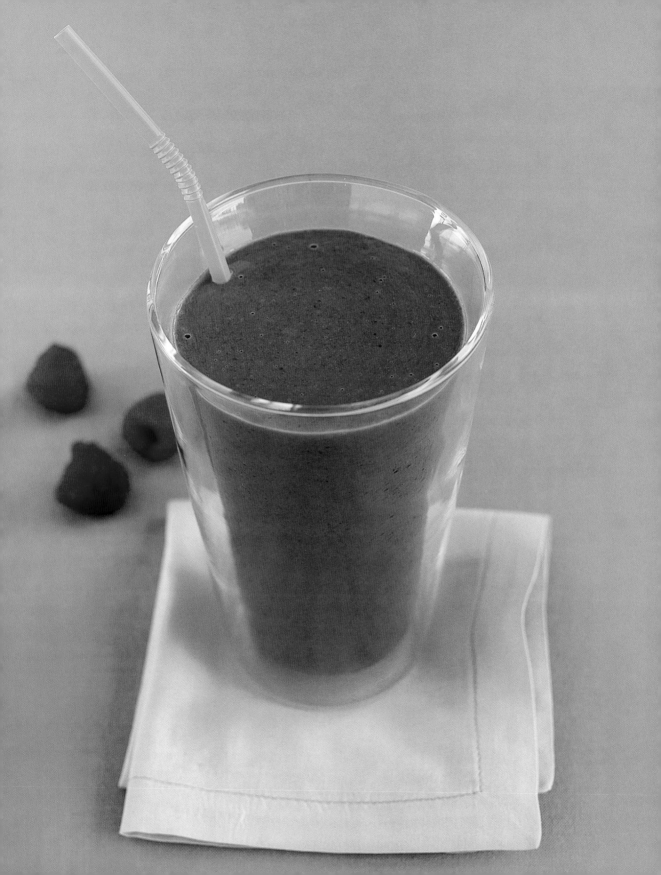

Soups & Sandwiches

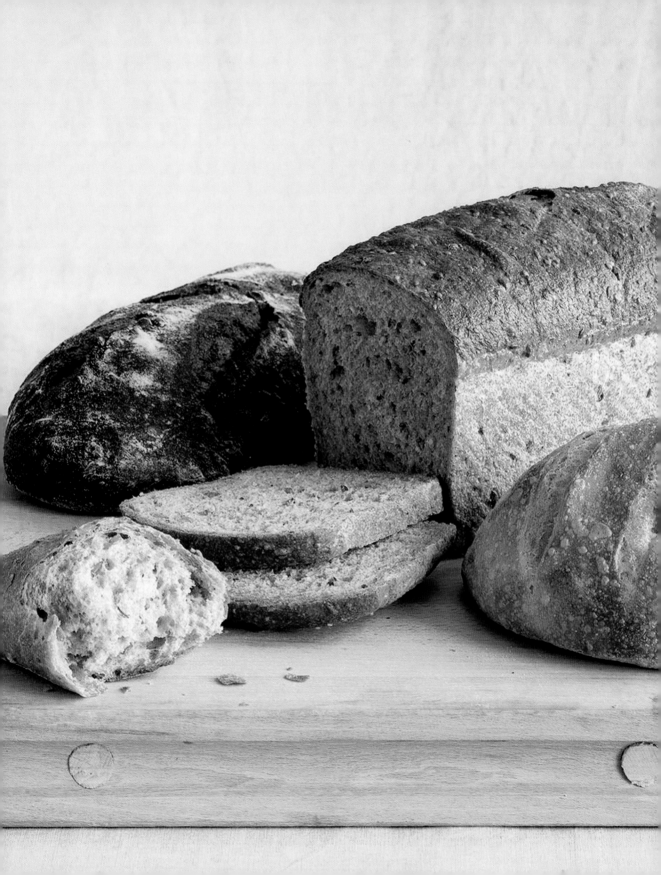

Three-Bean Soup with Canadian Bacon

Prep: *10 minutes* | **Cook:** *25 minutes* | **Total time:** *35 minutes* | **Makes:** *4 servings*

RS
3.5g

This superfast soup is the ultimate slimming, Resistant Starch–rich lunch. Enjoy it with a whole-grain roll.

1 tablespoon olive oil
1 cup diced onion
2 garlic cloves, chopped
1 large zucchini (about 2 cups), cut into small dice
1 quart low-sodium chicken stock
1 cup canned low-sodium cannellini beans, rinsed and drained
1 cup canned kidney beans, rinsed and drained
1 cup canned black beans, rinsed and drained
¼ teaspoon salt
¼ teaspoon pepper
2 slices (2 ounces) Canadian bacon, diced
  Cooking spray

1. Heat oil in a saucepan over medium-high heat.

2. Add onion and cook until soft, 6 minutes.

3. Add garlic and cook 1 minute.

4. Add zucchini and cook, stirring, 4 minutes.

5. Add stock, beans, salt, and pepper, and bring to a boil. Reduce heat, and simmer over very low heat until slightly thickened, 15 minutes.

6. While soup is simmering, cook bacon in a large nonstick skillet coated with cooking spray over medium-high heat until crisp, 3–5 minutes.

7. Divide soup among 4 bowls, and top each bowl with 1 tablespoon crisped bacon.

Serving size: 2 cups soup plus 1 tablespoon crisped Canadian bacon Calories 271; Fat 6.6g (sat 1.3g, mono 3.5g, poly 0.9g); Cholesterol 5mg; Protein 18g; Carbohydrate 38g; Sugars 6g; Fiber 11g; RS 3.5g; Sodium 504mg

TIP:
If you can't find fresh zucchini in winter, try substituting the same amount of chopped kale.

72

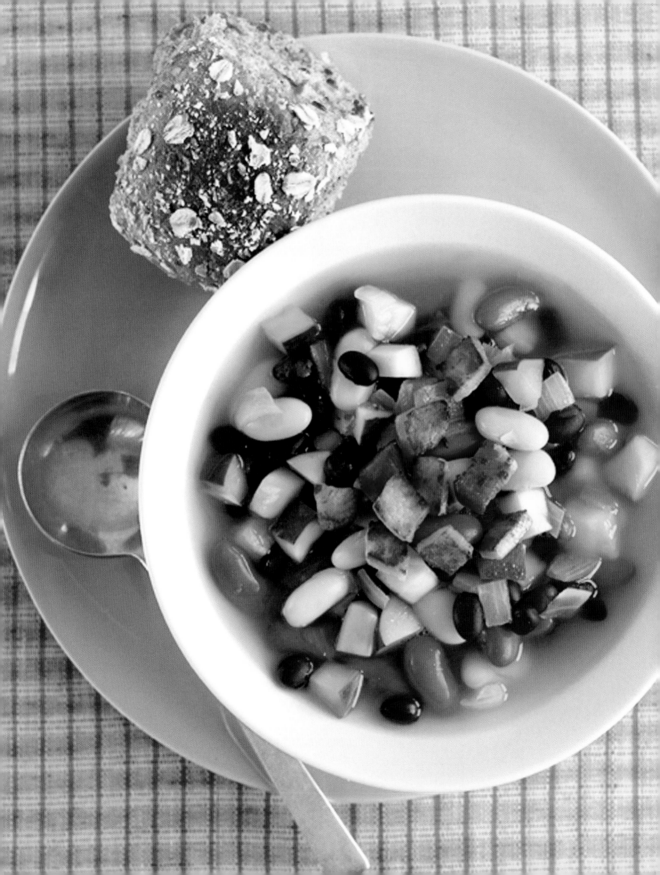

Hearty Chicken Posole Stew

Prep: *10 minutes* | **Cook:** *30 minutes* | **Total time:** *40 minutes* | **Makes:** *4 servings*

If you've never tried posole, you'll love adding this stew to your CarbLovers *menu! It's traditionally served in Mexico at Christmastime, but we think it's delicious anytime of year.*

1   tablespoon olive oil
1   small onion, chopped
2   cloves minced garlic
1   pound boneless, skinless chicken breast, cubed
¾   teaspoon cumin
½   teaspoon dried oregano
1   quart low-sodium chicken broth
1   (15-ounce) can fire-roasted tomatoes
1   (15-ounce) can hominy, rinsed and drained
1   tablespoon diced green chiles
½   teaspoon salt
¼   teaspoon pepper
    Fresh cilantro for garnish
    Tortilla chips (optional)

1. Heat oil in a medium saucepan over medium heat.

2. Add onion and cook until soft, about 7 minutes.

3. Add garlic and cook, stirring, 2 minutes.

4. Add chicken, cumin, and oregano, and cook, stirring, until just cooked through, 5 minutes.

5. Add broth, tomatoes, hominy, green chiles, salt, and pepper, and bring to a boil. Reduce heat, skimming foam from top of soup, and simmer, 10 minutes, until liquid has thickened slightly.

6. Divide soup among 4 bowls. Garnish with cilantro, and serve immediately with tortilla chips alongside, if desired.

Serving size: 2 cups stew Calories 303; Fat 8.5g (sat 1.8g, mono 4.3g, poly 1.7g); Cholesterol 63mg; Protein 30g; Carbohydrate 26g; Sugars 6g; Fiber 4g; RS 1.3g; Sodium 743mg

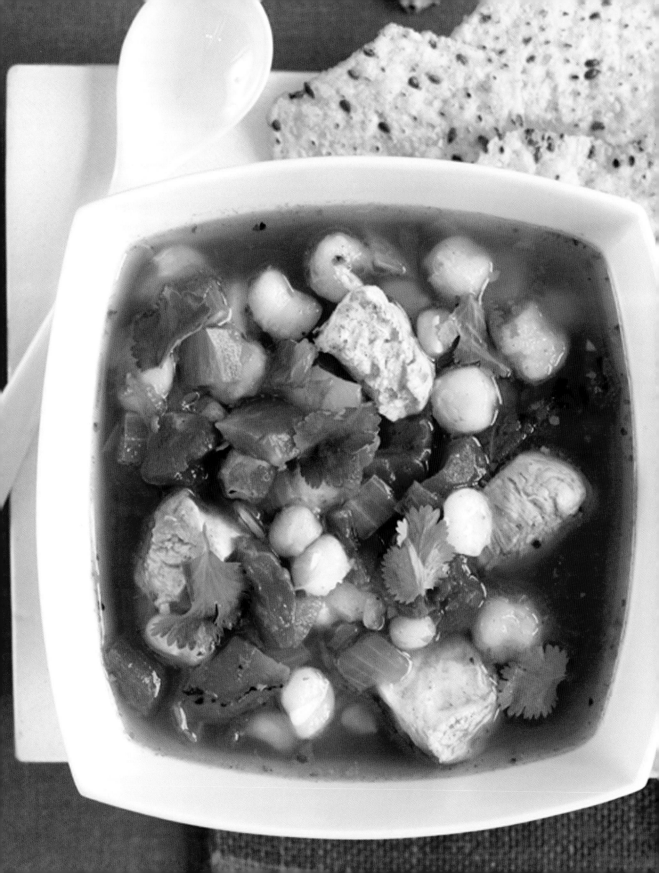

Chunky Tomato-Basil Soup with Pasta

Prep: 5 minutes | **Cook:** 20 minutes | **Total time:** 25 minutes | **Makes:** 4 servings

Take the chill out of a wintry day with this warming, savory soup. Pair it with half of our Grilled Cheese and Tomato on Rye (page 106) for a satisfying lunch or dinner.

1 tablespoon olive oil, plus more for serving if desired
1 small onion, chopped
2 tablespoons tomato paste
1 teaspoon sugar
⅛ teaspoon salt
1 (14.5-ounce) can low-sodium chicken broth
1 (28-ounce) can diced tomatoes in juice
1 garlic clove, peeled
2 large basil sprigs, leaves coarsely torn (1 cup) and stems reserved
2 ounces dry, small whole-wheat pasta (such as rotini, shells, or broken-up spaghetti)

1. Heat oil in a medium saucepan over medium heat. Add onion; cook, stirring occasionally, until tender, 5–7 minutes. Stir in tomato paste, sugar, and salt; cook 2 minutes. Stir in chicken broth, tomatoes and their juice, garlic, and basil stems; bring to a boil over high heat.

2. Add pasta; reduce heat to medium and simmer until pasta is tender and flavors are blended, about 10–12 minutes. Remove garlic clove and basil stems; discard. Serve pasta topped with basil leaves and a drizzle of olive oil.

Serving size: 1 cup Calories 156; Fat 4.1g (sat 0.7g, mono 2.5g, poly 0.5g); Cholesterol 2mg; Protein 6g; Carbohydrate 25g; Sugars 10g; Fiber 4g; RS 0.6g; Sodium 211mg

Creamy Clam and Corn Chowder

Prep: 20 minutes | *Cook:* 45 minutes | *Total time:* 65 minutes | *Makes:* 4 servings

Yes, you can enjoy creamy soup again. This rich-tasting, New England–style chowder is packed with Resistant Starch and delicious flavor.

2   teaspoons vegetable oil
2   ounces Canadian bacon, diced
1   medium onion, diced
2   stalks celery, diced
¼   cup dry white wine
3   cups low-fat milk (1%)
3   tablespoons flour
½   cup clam juice
1   bay leaf
1   large potato (12 ounces), peeled and diced
1   teaspoon Tabasco or other hot pepper sauce
¼   teaspoon pepper
1   cup fresh or frozen corn kernels, thawed
1   cup fresh chopped clams or 1 cup canned clams, rinsed and drained
2   tablespoons chopped fresh parsley

1. Heat oil in a medium saucepan over medium-high heat. Add bacon and cook, stirring, until crisped, 4–5 minutes. Add onion and celery and cook, stirring, until onion is softened and celery is cooked, about 6 minutes. Add wine and cook until most of the liquid is dissolved, 3 minutes.

2. Combine milk and flour in a large bowl and whisk until smooth. Add to the saucepan along with clam juice, ½ cup water, and bay leaf. Bring to a boil, reduce heat, and simmer, whisking, until thickened, 11 minutes. Add potato and cook until tender, about 12 minutes. Add Tabasco, pepper, corn, and clams, and simmer until clams and corn are cooked through, 4–5 minutes.

3. Divide among 4 bowls and garnish with parsley.

Serving size: 1½ cups chowder Calories 314; Fat 6.1g (sat 1.8g, mono 1.6g, poly 2g); Cholesterol 34mg; Protein 21g; Carbohydrate 42g; Sugars 13g; Fiber 3g; RS 1.1g; Sodium 739mg

French Onion Soup

Butternut Squash Soup

Cheesy
Garlic Bread

**Tortilla Chicken
Soup**

Butternut Squash Soup

Prep: 10 minutes | *Cook:* 25 minutes | *Total time:* 35 minutes | *Makes:* 4 servings

Creamy, comforting, and packed with beta-carotene, this soup makes a deliciously light lunch or a perfect start to a warming meal.

2   tablespoons olive oil, plus more
    for serving
1   medium onion, chopped
2   garlic cloves, chopped
½   teaspoon ground coriander
¼   teaspoon crushed red pepper, plus
    more for serving
1   tablespoon chopped fresh
    ginger
1   small butternut squash
    (1½ pounds), peeled, cut into
    1-inch cubes
1   quart low-sodium chicken broth
2   teaspoons fresh lemon juice

1. Heat oil in a large saucepan over medium heat. Add onion and garlic; cook, stirring occasionally, until tender, 6–8 minutes. Add coriander, crushed red pepper, and ginger; cook, stirring, 1 minute. Stir in squash, broth, and lemon juice; bring to a boil. Reduce heat to a simmer and cook 10 minutes or until squash is tender.

2. Working in batches, transfer soup to a blender and blend until smooth (or blend in the pan with an immersion blender). To serve, drizzle soup with a small amount of olive oil and sprinkle with crushed red pepper, if desired.

Serving size: About 1 cup Calories 148; Fat 7g (sat 1g, mono 4.9g, poly 0.8g); Cholesterol 0mg; Protein 4g; Carbohydrate 20g; Sugars 4g; Fiber 5g; RS 0g; Sodium 78mg

TIP:
Pour leftover broth into an ice cube tray, then seal the cubes in a freezer bag for later. Add them anytime you need a pop of flavor.

RS
1.4g

French Onion Soup

Prep: *5 minutes* | ***Cook:*** *50 minutes* | ***Total time:*** *55 minutes* | ***Makes:*** *4 servings*

This classic bistro soup is usually packed with sodium and fat, but we lightened up both without compromising flavor.

2   tablespoons vegetable oil
2   tablespoons butter
2½ pounds medium yellow onions
     (about 5), halved and thinly
     sliced
¼   cup Marsala wine (or sherry),
     divided
4   sprigs fresh thyme
2   (14.5-ounce) cans low-sodium
     beef broth
1   teaspoon red-wine vinegar
2   rectangular slices rye bread
     (about 3 ounces each), halved
2   thick slices low-fat Swiss cheese
     (about 2 ounces each), halved

1. Heat oil and butter in a Dutch oven or other large stockpot over medium heat. Add onions; cover and cook, stirring occasionally, until onions wilt and begin to brown on bottom of pan, about 20 minutes. Uncover and cook, stirring and adding Marsala 1 tablespoon at a time every 5 minutes, for 15 minutes. Stir in thyme, 3 cups water, broth, and vinegar; bring to a boil. Reduce heat to a simmer and cook 10 minutes or until flavors are blended.

2. Meanwhile, preheat broiler with rack in highest position. Arrange bread slices on a large rimmed baking sheet; top with cheese. Broil 2–3 minutes or until cheese is browned. Serve soup with cheese toasts.

Serving size: About 1⅔ cups Calories 429; Fat 16.9g (sat 5.8g, mono 4.6g, poly 5.3g); Cholesterol 25mg; Protein 19g; Carbohydrate 48g; Sugars 15g; Fiber 7g; RS 1.4g; Sodium 429mg

Tortilla Chicken Soup

Prep: *15 minutes* | **Cook:** *25 minutes* | **Total time:** *40 minutes* | **Makes:** *4 servings*

This soup is a spicy Mexican twist on the traditional winter warmer. We love the added crunch of the tortillas on top, plus the creamy avocado.

- 1 tablespoon olive oil, divided
- 1 small onion, chopped
- 2 teaspoons minced garlic
- 2 teaspoons seeded minced jalapeño peppers
- 1 teaspoon cumin
- ½ teaspoon salt, divided
- ½ teaspoon pepper
- 1 quart low-sodium chicken broth
- 1 (14.5-ounce) can low-sodium diced tomatoes
- 1 (12-ounce) can no-salt-added corn (about 1⅓ cups kernels), drained
- 1½ teaspoons mild hot sauce
- 2 (6-inch) corn tortillas
- 8 ounces white-meat rotisserie chicken (about 2 cups), skinned and shredded
- 1 small avocado, diced
- ¼ cup cilantro leaves
- 8 lime wedges

1. Preheat oven to 375°.

2. Heat 2 teaspoons oil in a medium saucepan over medium-high heat. Add onion and cook, stirring occasionally, until softened, 6 minutes. Add garlic, jalapeños, cumin, salt, and pepper, and cook 2 minutes. Add broth, tomatoes and their juice, corn, and hot sauce, and bring to a boil.

3. Reduce heat and simmer for 15 minutes. While soup is simmering, brush both sides of tortillas with remaining teaspoon oil. Using a pizza cutter or knife, cut tortillas into ¼-inch strips. Transfer to a baking sheet and bake until crisp and slightly browned, 7–8 minutes. Remove from oven and cool. When soup is done, divide among 4 bowls. Top with ¼ of the chicken, diced avocado, and tortilla strips, and a few cilantro leaves. Serve with lime wedges.

Serving size: 1½ cups soup Calories 306; Fat 11.9g (sat 1.8g, mono 6.9g, poly 1.7g); Cholesterol 50mg; Protein 23g; Carbohydrate 31g; Sugars 8g; Fiber 7g; RS 0.5g; Sodium 649mg

Cheesy Garlic Bread

Prep: 10 minutes | **Cook:** 15 minutes | **Total time:** 25 minutes | **Makes:** 8 servings

Who doesn't love garlic bread? Our crunchy version is excellent dunked in any of our soups or with saucy dishes like spaghetti and meatballs.

½ cup (2 ounces) grated Parmesan cheese
2 tablespoons olive oil
1 tablespoon softened butter
1 tablespoon reduced-fat mayonnaise
1 tablespoon minced garlic
¼ teaspoon salt
¼ teaspoon pepper
¼ cup minced parsley
1 (12-inch) French bread loaf, split

1. Preheat oven to 400°.

2. Combine Parmesan, oil, butter, mayonnaise, garlic, salt, and pepper, and spread evenly on both bread halves. Wrap bread loosely in aluminum foil and place on a baking sheet. Bake until golden brown and crust is crisp, 13–15 minutes. Remove bread halves from oven and cut each (using a serrated bread knife) into 4 (3-inch) pieces.

Serving size: 1 (3-inch) piece bread Calories 144; Fat 7.2g (sat 2.3g, mono 3.4g, poly 0.8g); Cholesterol 9mg; Protein 4g; Carbohydrate 15g; Sugars 1g; Fiber 1g; RS 0.3g; Sodium 364mg

RS 1.9g

Mexican Mole Chili

Prep: 15 minutes | *Cook:* 45 minutes | *Total time:* 1 hour | *Makes:* 6 servings

This hearty bowl has some kick from two different types of chili powder, plus crushed red pepper. And it's fiber-packed! Make a batch for your Super Bowl bash or post-sledding party.

- 1 tablespoon olive oil
- 1 large onion, chopped
- 1 tablespoon minced garlic
- 1 pound lean ground beef or bison
- 3 tablespoons unsweetened cocoa
- 1 tablespoon chili powder
- 1 teaspoon cumin
- 1 teaspoon chipotle chile powder
- ¾ teaspoon salt
- ½ teaspoon pepper
- ½ teaspoon crushed red pepper
- 2 green bell peppers, seeded and chopped
- 2 (15-ounce) cans low-sodium diced tomatoes in juice
- 1 (15-ounce) can kidney beans
- 1 (15-ounce) can black beans
- ¼ cup chopped fresh cilantro
- 2 tablespoons diced red onion
  Light sour cream (optional)

1. Heat oil in a large stockpot over medium-high heat. Add onion and cook until softened, 6–7 minutes. Add garlic and cook 1 minute. Add beef and cook, breaking up with a spoon, until just cooked through, 5 minutes. Add cocoa, chili powder, cumin, chipotle powder, salt, pepper, and crushed red pepper, and cook for 1 minute until fragrant. Add bell peppers, tomatoes, and beans, and bring to a boil. Cover, reduce heat, and simmer until liquid is absorbed, 40–45 minutes.

2. Divide among 6 bowls and garnish with cilantro, onion, and sour cream, if desired.

Serving size: 1⅓ cups Calories 355; Fat 11.1g (sat 3.6g, mono 5g, poly 0.9g); Cholesterol 49mg; Protein 27g; Carbohydrate 38g; Sugars 7g; Fiber 11g; RS 1.9g; Sodium 624mg

> **TIP:**
> Our perfectly sized Mini Corn and Feta Muffins are an ideal partner for this spicy chili. Find the recipe on page 212.

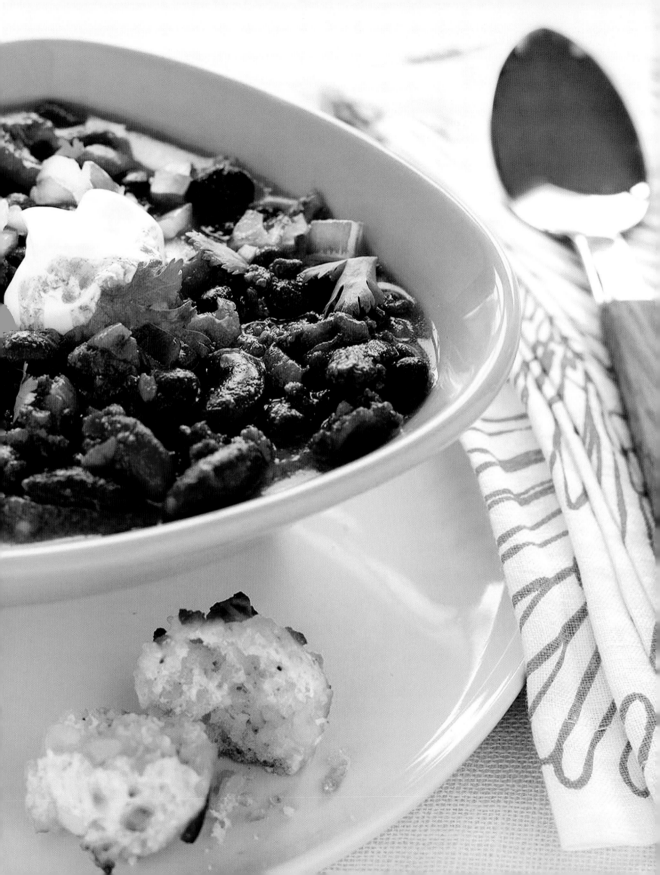

Chicken Noodle Soup with Fall Vegetables

Prep: *5 minutes* | **Cook:** *20 minutes* | **Total time:** *25 minutes* | **Makes:** *4 servings*

Other than a hug from Mom, nothing makes you feel as good as a warm bowl of homemade chicken soup. This healthy variation gets a touch of sweetness from the parsnips and nutmeg.

1	tablespoon olive oil
1	garlic clove, finely chopped
1	small onion, chopped
1	celery rib, cut into ½-inch pieces
1	parsnip, halved and sliced crosswise
1	carrot, halved and sliced crosswise
1	quart reduced-sodium chicken broth
2	boneless, skinless chicken breasts (about 1 pound total)
¼	teaspoon kosher salt
¼	teaspoon freshly ground black pepper
¼	teaspoon freshly grated nutmeg
4	sprigs fresh thyme
1½	cups (6 ounces) whole-wheat medium egg noodles

1. Heat oil in a large stockpot over medium-low heat. Add garlic, onion, celery, parsnip, and carrot; cook, stirring occasionally, until vegetables are crisp-tender, 5–7 minutes. Add broth, chicken, salt, pepper, nutmeg, and thyme. Bring to a boil; reduce heat to medium and simmer 10–15 minutes or until chicken is cooked through. Remove chicken; set aside.

2. Return broth mixture to a boil. Add noodles; simmer 5–8 minutes or until tender. Pull chicken apart into thin strips; return to soup and serve.

Serving size: 1¼ cups Calories 343; Fat 8.7g (sat 1.6g, mono 4g, poly 1.4g); Cholesterol 103mg; Protein 31g; Carbohydrate 34g; Sugars 3g; Fiber 3g; RS 1.7g; Sodium 729mg

TIP:
Have a hot bowl of chicken soup ready in minutes by making extra and freezing it. Chill first, then place portions in freezer-safe containers. Thaw, heat, and enjoy!

RS
0.6g

Apple, Gouda, and Turkey Wrap with Bacon

Prep: 5 minutes | *Cook:* 10 minutes | *Total time:* 15 minutes | *Makes:* 4 servings

Crispy, sweet apples and salty Gouda cheese are a natural pairing. Add in some turkey and a little bacon, and you've got one delicious wrap.

4 slices center-cut bacon
4 (10-inch) whole-wheat wraps
3 ounces Gouda, sliced
4 ounces thinly sliced roasted deli turkey
1 medium crisp apple (such as Gala), thinly sliced
1 cup mesclun greens

1. Heat a large nonstick skillet over medium heat; add bacon. Cook, turning often, until bacon is crispy, 6–8 minutes. Drain on paper towels, and set aside.

2. Arrange wraps on a clean work surface. Place ¼ of the cheese and turkey slices in the center of each wrap. Top turkey with ¼ of the apple slices, 1 slice of the cooled bacon, and ¼ cup of the salad greens; roll wraps, folding in sides, to enclose filling.

Serving size: 1 wrap Calories 256; Fat 12.5g (sat 4.9g, mono 4.6g, poly 1.5g); Cholesterol 43mg; Protein 23g; Carbohydrate 26g; Sugars 7g; Fiber 13g; RS 0.6g; Sodium 734mg

Chicken Parmesan Hero

Prep: 20 minutes | **Cook:** 30 minutes | **Total time:** 50 minutes | **Makes:** 4 servings

☺

Zesty homemade marinara sauce, gooey cheese, and crispy chicken meld together in this dream of a sandwich. Save time by using store-bought whole wheat bread crumbs.

4 slices whole-wheat bread
¾ teaspoon paprika, divided
½ teaspoon garlic powder
1 tablespoon olive oil
1 small onion (1 cup), diced
2 cloves minced garlic
1 (26.46-ounce) box of chopped tomatoes (such as Pomi)
½ cup all-purpose flour
½ teaspoon black pepper
3 egg whites, whisked
4 (4–5 ounce) boneless, skinless chicken breasts, pounded to ½-inch thickness
Olive oil cooking spray
2 whole-grain rolls (5–6 inches), split
1 cup baby spinach leaves
¾ cup shredded part-skim mozzarella cheese

1. Preheat oven to 375°.

2. Process bread in a food processor until crumbs form, about 20 seconds. Toast crumbs on a baking sheet until golden, tossing occasionally, 7–8 minutes. Remove from oven and cool. Transfer to a shallow dish; toss with ½ teaspoon paprika and garlic powder. Set aside.

3. Heat oil in a medium saucepan over medium-high heat. Add onion and cook until soft and translucent, 6–7 minutes. Add garlic and cook 1 minute. Add tomatoes and their juices and bring to a boil. Reduce heat and simmer until sauce thickens slightly, 10 minutes. Remove from heat; reserve. In a resealable plastic bag, combine flour, remaining paprika, and pepper. Shake each piece of chicken in flour mixture, then dip in egg, then in reserved bread crumbs, shaking off excess.

4. Place chicken in a baking dish and coat each side with cooking spray. Bake until cooked though and browned, about 12–13 minutes.

5. Place rolls on a baking sheet. Spoon about ¼ cup marinara sauce onto one side of a roll and top with ¼ cup spinach leaves. Top with a breaded cutlet, an additional ¼ cup marinara sauce, and 3 tablespoons mozzarella. Return to oven until cheese is melted, about 5 minutes.

Serving size: ½ roll, ½ cup marinara sauce, 1 cutlet, ¼ cup spinach leaves, 3 tablespoons mozzarella cheese Calories 563; Fat 14.9g (sat 4.4g, mono 5.4g, poly 3.2g); Cholesterol 90mg; Protein 48g; Carbohydrate 58g; Sugars 5g; Fiber 11g; RS 0.8g; Sodium 552mg

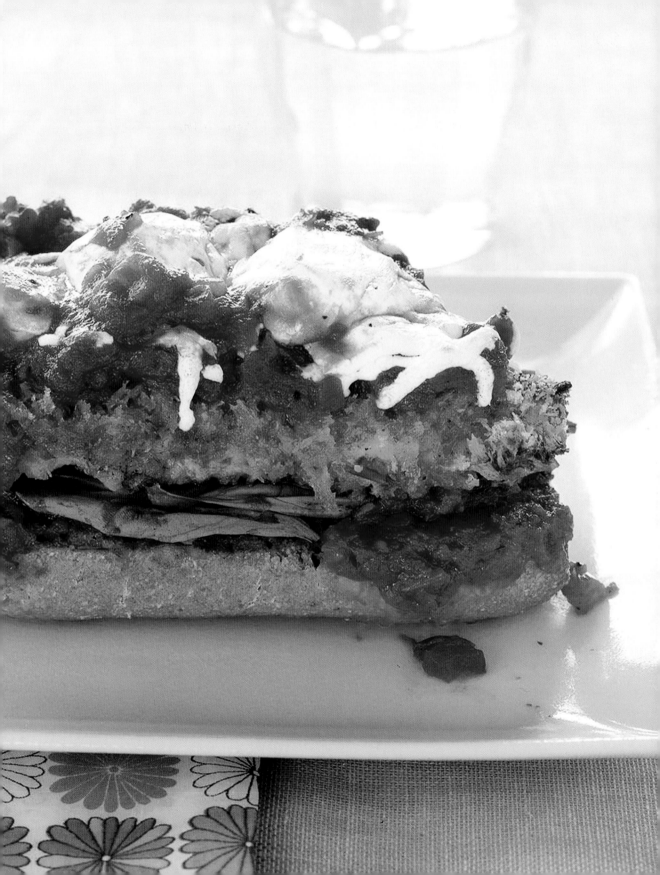

RS
2.2g

CarbLovers Club Sandwich

Prep: 15 minutes | **Cook:** 10 minutes | **Total time:** 25 minutes | **Makes:** 4 servings

Bite into the amazing combination of creamy avocado, salty bacon, and cool tomato. Perfection on a plate!

¾ cup canned low-sodium cannellini beans, rinsed and drained
2 cloves roasted garlic (such as Christopher Ranch brand)
1 tablespoon olive oil
¼ teaspoon salt
¼ teaspoon pepper
12 slices thin whole-wheat bread, toasted
8 leaves butter lettuce
1 beefsteak tomato, sliced
1 avocado, pitted and sliced
8 slices turkey bacon, cooked according to package directions and drained on paper towels

1. Mash beans, garlic, oil, salt, and pepper with a fork and reserve.

2. Arrange 4 bread slices on a work surface. Spread 3 tablespoons white-bean mixture on each slice of bread.

3. Top with 2 lettuce leaves and 2 tomato slices.

4. Layer another slice of bread on each sandwich, and top each with 4 avocado slices and 2 turkey bacon slices. Top with last piece of bread.

5. Halve sandwiches diagonally, and secure with toothpicks.

Serving size: 1 sandwich Calories 412; Fat 17.5g (sat 2.4g, mono 10.1g, poly 3.6g); Cholesterol 14mg; Protein 16g; Carbohydrate 47g; Sugars 5g; Fiber 12g; RS 2.2g; Sodium 572mg

TIP:
Make extra bean spread when you're whipping up this sandwich, and use it as a dip for fresh vegetables and tortilla chips.

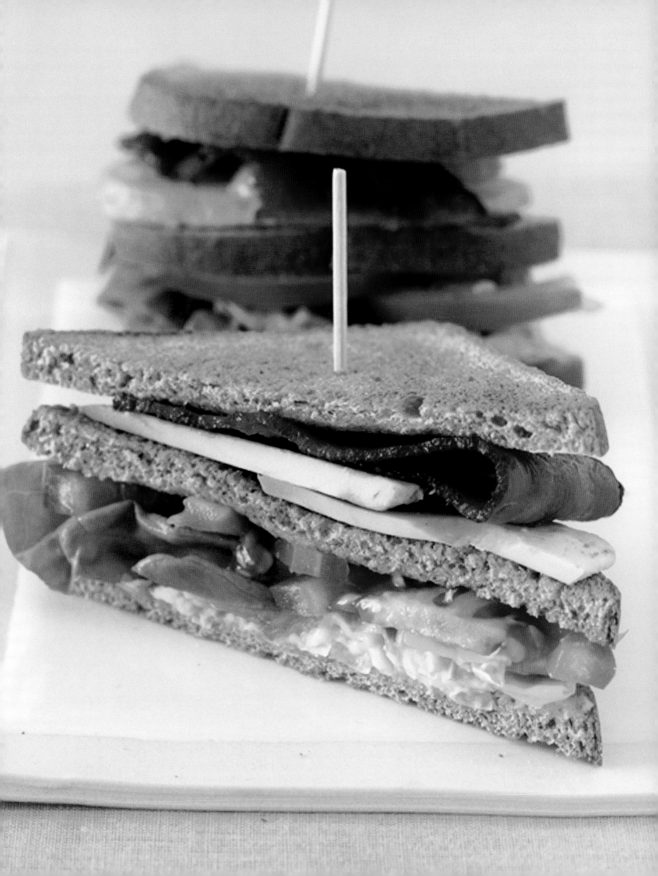

RS
6.9g

Stacked Deli Sandwiches with Homemade Coleslaw

Prep: *5 minutes* | **Cook:** *15 minutes* | **Total time:** *20 minutes* | **Makes:** *4 servings*

These impressive (and Resistant Starch–loaded!) sandwiches are stacked to the hilt with tasty ingredients. Serve them at your next book club meeting or picnic.

FOR RUSSIAN DRESSING:

- 3 tablespoons light mayonnaise
- 3 tablespoons reduced-fat sour cream
- 1 tablespoon ketchup
- 1 teaspoon red wine vinegar
- 1 teaspoon chopped dill pickles

FOR COLESLAW:

- 4 cups bagged coleslaw mix
- 2 cups shredded red cabbage
- 2 tablespoons apple cider vinegar
- 1 tablespoon vegetable oil
- 2 teaspoons lightly toasted caraway seeds
- 2 teaspoons Dijon mustard

FOR SANDWICHES:

- 8 (1½-ounce) slices dark pumpernickel bread
- 6 ounces thinly sliced roast beef
- 6 ounces thinly sliced fresh roasted turkey breast
- 4 (½-ounce) slices reduced-fat Swiss cheese
- 1 large beefsteak tomato, cut into 8 slices

MAKE RUSSIAN DRESSING:

1. Whisk together mayonnaise, sour cream, ketchup, red wine vinegar, and pickles in a small bowl; reserve.

MAKE COLESLAW:

2. Toss coleslaw mix, cabbage, cider vinegar, oil, caraway, and mustard in a large bowl; reserve.

MAKE SANDWICHES:

3. Spread about 1 tablespoon Russian dressing on each slice of bread. Top 4 slices with 1½ ounces roast beef and a tomato slice. Add 1½ ounce turkey, then another tomato slice. Top with cheese. Finish with second slice of bread, dressing side down. Serve with 1 cup coleslaw, either on the sandwich or alongside (you'll have some leftover).

Serving size: 1 sandwich plus about 1 cup coleslaw
Calories 497; Fat 15g (sat 4.8g, mono 3.4g, poly 4.5g); Cholesterol 76mg; Protein 36g; Carbohydrate 56g; Sugars 15g; Fiber 6g; RS 6.9g; Sodium 744mg

TIP:
If you're packing these for a picnic or road trip, leave off the coleslaw and dressing. Add to the sandwiches before serving.

Curried Tuna Salad Sandwiches

Prep: 15 minutes | *Total time:* 15 minutes | *Makes:* 4 servings

Spice up ordinary tuna with a hint of curry and the unexpected sweetness of raisins.

¼ cup light mayonnaise

1½ teaspoons curry powder

¼ teaspoon salt

½ teaspoon pepper

2 5-ounce cans water-packed light tuna, drained

2 ribs minced celery (about ⅔ cup)

½ cup chopped water chestnuts

3 tablespoons finely minced red onion

3 tablespoons golden raisins

4 lettuce leaves

8 tomato slices

8 slices whole-wheat bread, toasted

1. Whisk together mayonnaise, curry powder, salt and pepper in a medium bowl. Add tuna, celery, water chestnuts, onion, and raisins and mix well.

2. Place a lettuce leaf and 2 tomato slices on a piece of toasted bread. Add about ⅔ cup tuna mixture and top with another slice of bread. Serve immediately.

Serving size: 1 sandwich Calories 433; Fat 10.8g (sat 1.7g, mono 2.5g, poly 5.7g); Cholesterol 27mg; Protein 27g; Carbohydrate 60g; Sugars 10g; Fiber 8g; RS 1g; Sodium 621mg

Falafel Pita with Tahini Sauce

Prep: *15 minutes* | **Cook:** *10 minutes* | **Total time:** *25 minutes* | **Makes:** *6 servings*

Even meat eaters will love these veggie burgers! The patties are a spin on falafel, but instead of deep-frying, we give them a light pan-fry. And since the recipe takes less than 30 minutes, it's great for a quick and tasty weeknight meal.

⅔   cup uncooked bulgur
1   cup boiling water
1   (15-ounce) can garbanzo beans, rinsed and drained
1   large egg white
½   cup packed fresh parsley leaves
¼   cup packed fresh mint leaves
1   garlic clove, roughly chopped
¼   teaspoon cayenne pepper
1   teaspoon ground cumin
¼   teaspoon salt
¼   teaspoon pepper
1   tablespoon olive oil
¼   cup tahini
2   tablespoons fresh lemon juice
6   (6-inch) pitas
4   cups torn lettuce
1   cup roasted red peppers

1. Combine bulgur and boiling water in a medium bowl. Cover and let stand 10 minutes or until just warm; drain. Transfer to a food processor with beans, egg white, parsley, mint, garlic, cayenne, cumin, salt, and pepper. Form mixture into 6 (approximately 3-inch, about ⅓ cup each) patties and place on a large plate. Refrigerate 20 minutes or until firm.

2. Heat oil in a large nonstick skillet over medium-high heat. Cook falafels until browned and heated through, 3 minutes per side. Transfer to a plate.

3. Whisk together tahini, lemon juice, and ¼ cup water in a medium bowl until light and fluffy. Serve in pitas with lettuce, roasted red peppers, and falafels.

Serving size: 1 burger, 2 tablespoons tahini mixture
Calories 396; Fat 10g (sat 1.4g, mono 4g, poly 3.6g); Cholesterol 0mg; Protein 15g; Carbohydrate 64g; Sugars 5g; Fiber 10g; RS 2.4g; Sodium 602mg

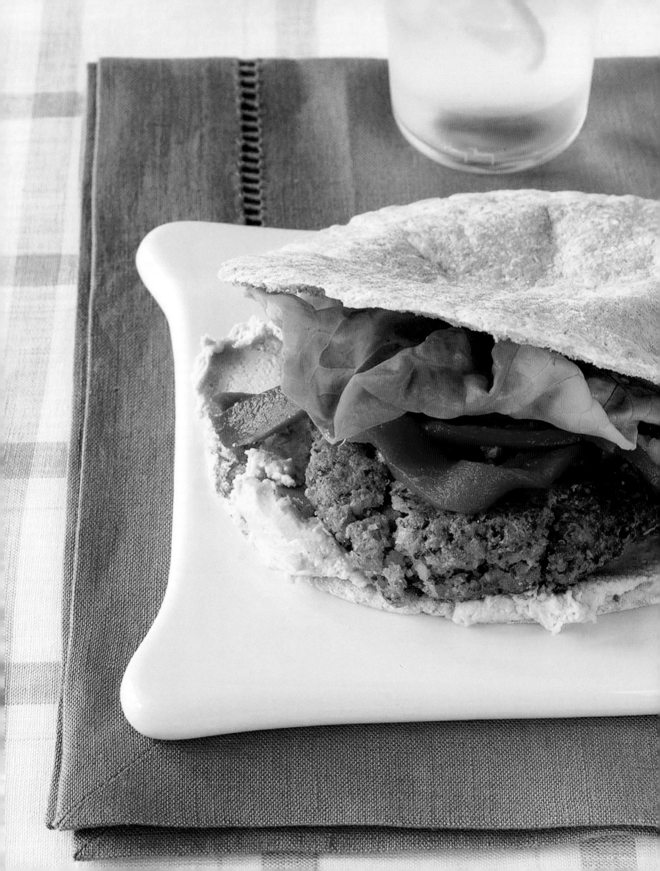

Teriyaki Steak Sandwich

Prep: 20 minutes | **Cook:** 15 minutes | **Total time:** 35 minutes | **Makes:** 4 servings

Looking for a sandwich with a bit more flair? This is it! The delicious teriyaki flavor makes this great for lunch or dinner, and the 26 grams of protein and 15 grams of fiber will keep you satisfied for hours.

FOR TERIYAKI SAUCE:

- 2 tablesoons low-sodium soy sauce
- 3 tablespoons light brown sugar
- 1 tablespoon minced fresh ginger
- 2 teaspoons minced garlic
- 1 teaspoon cornstarch
- 1 teaspoon sesame oil
- ½ teaspoon chile-garlic sauce (such as Sriracha)

FOR SANDWICH:

- 4 teaspoons vegetable oil, divided
- ¾ pound lean sirloin steak, very thinly sliced
- 2 bunches scallions, trimmed, cut into 2-inch lengths, whites and greens separated (about 2 cups)
- 4 cups sliced shiitake mushrooms (6 ounces)
- 1 cup snow peas (4 ounces)
- 4 10-inch whole-wheat wraps

MAKE TERIYAKI SAUCE:

1. Whisk together soy sauce, ¼ cup water, sugar, ginger, garlic, cornstarch, sesame oil, and chile-garlic sauce in a bowl. Reserve.

MAKE SANDWICH:

2. Heat 2 teaspoons oil in a large skillet over medium-high heat. Add steak and cook until browned and just cooked through, 2–3 minutes per side. Transfer steak (with its juices) to a bowl. Add remaining 2 teaspoons oil to pan, then add scallion whites and cook, stirring, until charred, 2 minutes. Add mushrooms and cook until softened, 3–4 minutes. Return beef to pan, add scallion greens, snow peas, and teriyaki sauce and cook until heated through and entire mixture is thickened, 2–3 minutes.

3. Place about ¾ cup mixture in middle of wrap and wrap tightly. Slice in half and serve warm.

Serving size: 1 wrap and ¾ cup mixture Calories 342; Fat 15.1g (sat 2.8g, mono 5.3g, poly 4.9g); Cholesterol 41mg; Protein 26g; Carbohydrate 39g; Sugars 15g; Fiber 15g; RS 0.6g; Sodium 640mg

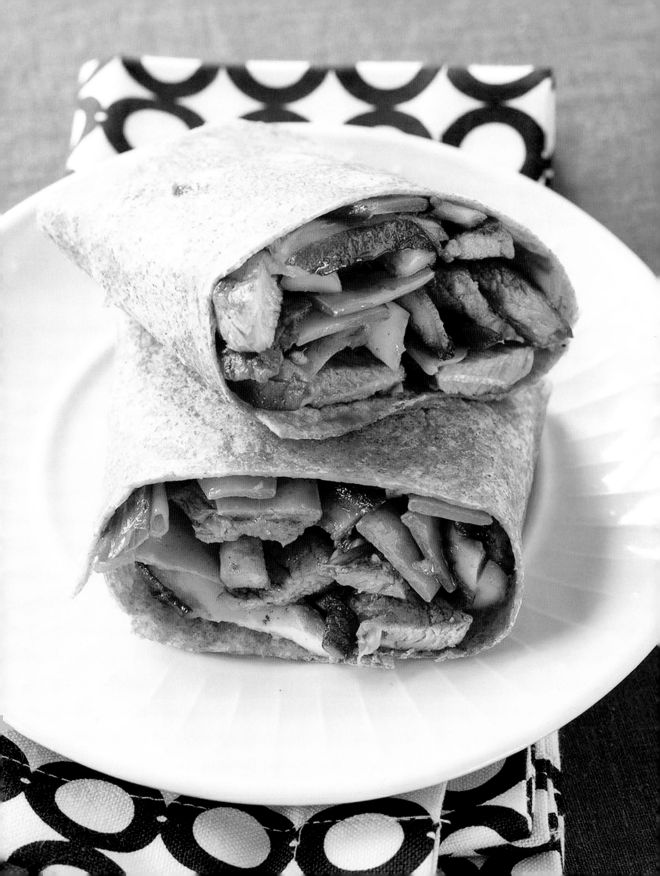

RS
2.9g

Roast Beef Pumpernickel Sandwich with Roasted Red Pepper, Arugula, and Goat Cheese

Prep: *10 minutes* | **Total time:** *10 minutes* | **Makes:** *4 servings*

Juicy deli sandwiches have probably been on your "no-no" list for years. Ours lets you indulge without the bulge, and has almost 3 grams of Resistant Starch!

3 ounces goat cheese, softened

8 slices pumpernickel bread

4 lettuce leaves

12 ounces thinly sliced lean roast beef

4 jarred roasted red peppers (2 ounces each), rinsed, drained, patted dry, and halved

4 teaspoons balsamic vinegar

1. Spread goat cheese on 4 slices of bread.

2. Arrange 1 lettuce leaf on each cheese-topped bread slice, then layer each with 3 ounces roast beef.

3. Top with red peppers, drizzle with vinegar, and cover with remaining bread slices. Serve.

Serving size: 1 sandwich Calories 380; Fat 11.4g (sat 5.1g, mono 3.7g, poly 1.1g); Cholesterol 74mg; Protein 33g; Carbohydrate 38g; Sugars 3g; Fiber 4g; RS 2.9g; Sodium 653mg

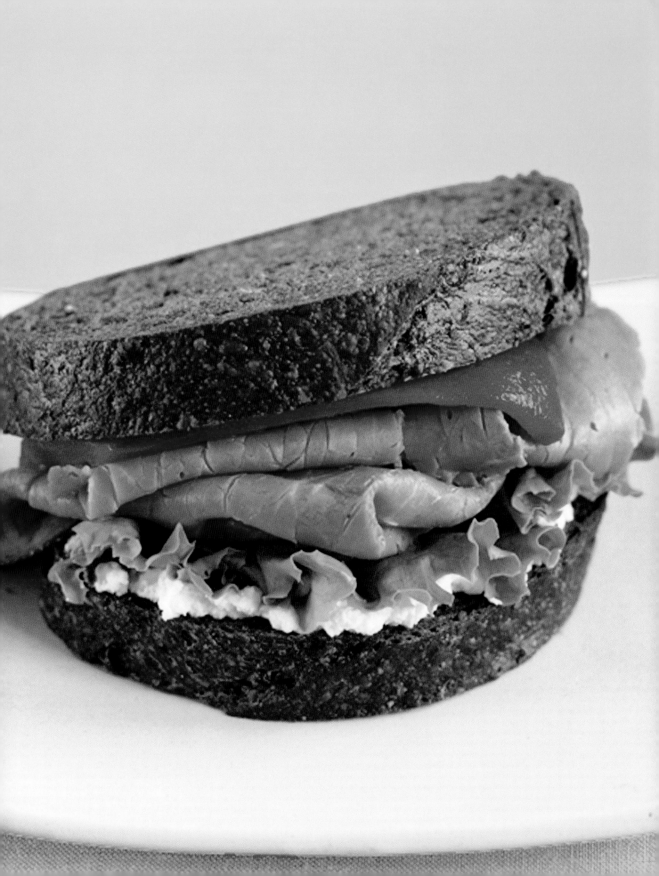

Tuna and White Bean Crostino

Prep: *2 minutes* | **Cook:** *3 minutes* | **Total time:** *5 minutes* | **Makes:** *4 servings*

Got 5 minutes? Then you can whip up this savory, Resistant Starch–packed crostino.

1 (5-ounce) can tuna in olive oil,
   drained and flaked
1 (15-ounce) can white beans,
   drained
1 tablespoon chopped fresh parsley
2 tablespoons fresh lemon juice
¼ teaspoon kosher salt
¼ teaspoon freshly ground black
   pepper
4 slices whole-wheat country bread
   (about 2 ounces each)
2 ounces Fontina cheese, coarsely
   grated

Preheat broiler with rack in highest position. Stir together tuna, beans, parsley, lemon juice, salt, and pepper in a medium bowl. Arrange bread on a baking sheet; divide tuna salad among bread slices. Top crostino with cheese; broil until golden, 2–3 minutes.

Serving size: 1 crostino Calories 394; Fat 10.7g (sat 3.8g, mono 3g, poly 3g); Cholesterol 23mg; Protein 26g; Carbohydrate 50g; Sugars 3g; Fiber 8g; RS 3.9; Sodium 754mg

> **TIP:**
> Convert this from a lunch to an appetizer by using slices of toasted baguette. Mash the beans for a creamier texture.

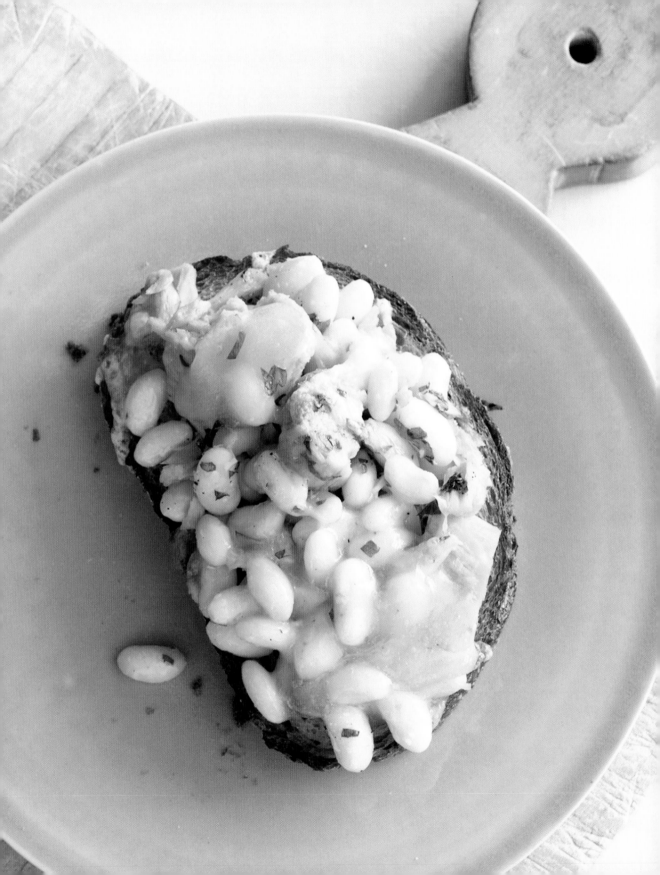

RS
2.7g

Black Bean, Avocado, Brown Rice, and Chicken Wrap

Prep: *15 minutes* | **Total time:** *15 minutes* | **Makes:** *4 servings*

Superfast and satisfying, this wrap is one of our favorites. It's also great for a make-your-own-burrito night with the kids. Just put all the ingredients in little bowls, and let them get creative.

½   teaspoon salt
¼   teaspoon freshly ground black pepper
1⅓ cup low-sodium black beans, rinsed and drained
1   teaspoon chili powder
½   teaspoon cumin
¼   teaspoon crushed red pepper
4   (10-inch) whole-wheat wraps
1⅓ cups cooked brown rice
8   ounces grilled chicken breast, sliced
1   small carrot, shredded (about 1 cup)
½   avocado, pitted and diced
    Hot sauce for serving (optional)
1   plum tomato, seeded and chopped (½ cup)

1. Place salt, pepper, beans, chili powder, cumin, and crushed red pepper in a small bowl and toss to combine.

2. Place one wrap on a clean work surface. Spoon ⅓ cup rice onto bottom of wrap. Add ⅓ cup bean mixture, 2 ounces chicken, and ¼ cup carrot, then top with about 1 tablespoon avocado and 2 tablespoons tomato.

3. Seal wrap, slice in half, and serve immediately with hot sauce on the side, if desired.

Serving size: 1 wrap Calories 425; Fat 9g (sat 1.3g, mono 3.4g, poly 1.2g); Cholesterol 48mg; Protein 31g; Carbohydrate 60g; Sugars 7g; Fiber 12g; RS 2.7g; Sodium 636mg

ASK CARBLOVERS

Q: **I am a vegetarian. How do I modify the *CarbLovers* diet to fit my needs?**

A: Since it's mainly built around grains, beans, and vegetables, *CarbLovers* is perfect for vegetarians. And you can always make tweaks to recipes like the one above, substituting firm tofu for the chicken, or adding a side of beans to grain dishes.

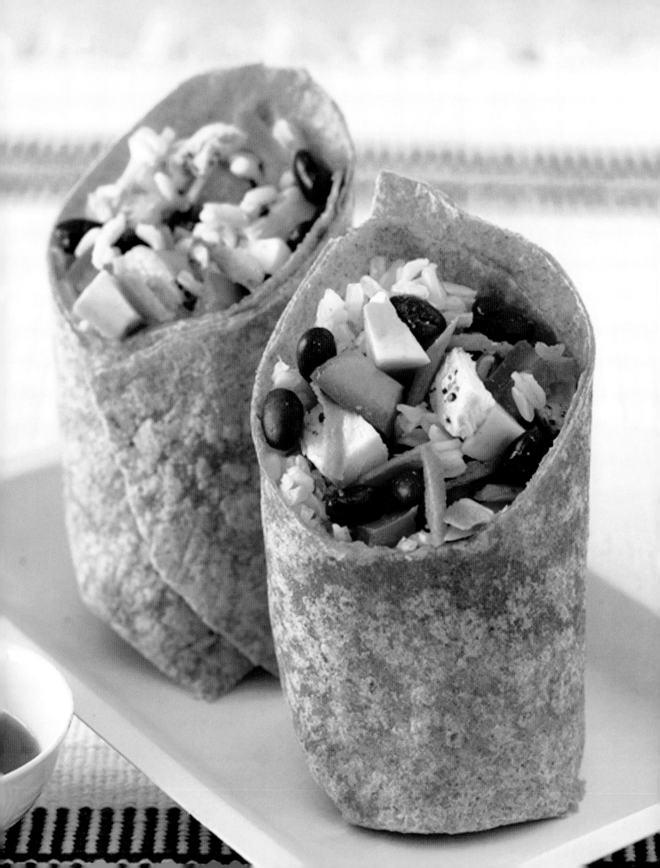

Roasted Corn and Black Bean Burrito

Prep: 10 minutes | **Cook:** 5 minutes | **Total time:** 15 minutes | **Makes:** 4 servings

Black beans are an amazing source of Resistant Starch and fiber (this recipe has 20 grams!). But not only is this burrito filling and healthy, it's also packed with flavor from the fresh lime juice and cilantro.

1 cup corn kernels, thawed and patted dry
1 (15-ounce) can black beans, rinsed and drained
¼ cup finely diced red onion
¼ teaspoon chipotle chile powder
1 tablespoon fresh lime juice
1 teaspoon olive oil
¼ cup chopped cilantro
¼ teaspoon salt
¼ teaspoon pepper
4 (10-inch) whole-wheat tortillas
1 cup hot cooked white rice
1 cup shredded romaine lettuce
½ cup shredded Monterey Jack cheese

1. Heat a large cast-iron or other heavy skillet over high heat until very hot, 3 minutes. Add corn; cook, stirring occasionally, until charred, about 3 minutes. Remove from heat and toss with next 8 ingredients (through pepper).

2. Spread ¼ cup cooked rice over the bottom half of a tortilla, leaving a 1-inch border. Top rice with a heaping ½ cup corn and bean mixture, ¼ cup shredded lettuce, and 2 tablespoons cheese; roll up. Repeat with remaining ingredients. Slice each burrito in half, and serve.

Serving size: 1 burrito with ½ cup corn and bean mixture Calories 331; Fat 9.3g (sat 3g, mono 3.7g, poly 1.6g); Cholesterol 13mg; Protein 21g; Carbohydrate 56g; Sugars 3g; Fiber 20g; RS 2.3g; Sodium 705mg

> **TIP:**
> Boost the Resistant Starch in this recipe even higher by using brown rice instead of white.

Saucy Turkey Meatball Sub

Prep: 25 minutes | *Cook:* 25 minutes | *Total time:* 50 minutes | *Makes:* 4 servings

We've taken a huge diet no-no and turned it into a "Yes, please!" This sub sandwich will satisfy even your most die-hard meat eaters. Serve with plenty of napkins.

2   cups marinara sauce
1   pound ground turkey
¼   cup fresh bread crumbs
⅓   cup grated Pecorino Romano cheese, divided
¾   cup finely grated carrot
¼   cup finely chopped onion
2   cloves garlic, minced
3   tablespoons minced fresh parsley
2   tablespoons ketchup
¼   teaspoon salt
¼   teaspoon pepper
      Cooking spray
4   whole-wheat hot dog buns, split and lightly toasted

1. Place marinara sauce in a medium saucepan and keep warm on low.

2. Combine turkey, bread crumbs, ¼ cup cheese, carrot, onion, garlic, parsley, ketchup, salt, and pepper in a bowl and mix with clean hands until well incorporated. Using slightly wet hands, form into 16 equal-size meatballs. Heat a large nonstick skillet coated with cooking spray over medium-high heat; brown meatballs on all sides, about 5–6 minutes.

3. Add meatballs to sauce, increase heat to medium, and simmer until meatballs have absorbed some of the sauce and are heated through, 10–15 minutes. Spoon 4 meatballs and some sauce onto a bun and sprinkle with 1 tablespoon cheese.

Serving size: 1 sub Calories 431; Fat 15g (sat 4.4g, mono 3g, poly 2.5g); Cholesterol 88mg; Protein 34g; Carbohydrate 43g; Sugars 12g; Fiber 5g; RS 1.1g; Sodium 1,131mg

TIP:
If you're on a low-sodium diet, use no-salt-added marinara and skip the cheese and added salt.

RS
1.8g

Grilled Cheese and Tomato on Rye

Prep: *5 minutes* | **Cook:** *6 minutes* | **Total time:** *11 minutes* | **Makes:** *4 servings*

Sometimes the simplest ingredients can be the most satisfying. That's the case with this toasty spin on grilled cheese. Enjoy it with a piece of fresh fruit for a filling lunch.

Cooking spray
2 tablespoons whole grain mustard
8 slices rye bread
8 ounces reduced-fat Cheddar
cheese, sliced
1 beefsteak tomato, sliced

1. Heat a large nonstick skillet coated with cooking spray over medium-high heat.

2. Spread ½ tablespoon mustard on each of 4 slices of bread, then top each with 2 slices cheese and 1 slice tomato. Top with remaining bread slices.

3. Place sandwiches in pan; place another pan on top of the sandwiches.

4. Cook until bottoms of sandwiches are browned, 2–3 minutes. Flip and cook, 2–3 minutes, until bread is golden and cheese is melted.

Serving size: 1 sandwich Calories 328; Fat 12.5g (sat 6.6g, mono 3.6g, poly 0.9g); Cholesterol 32mg; Protein 22g; Carbohydrate 31g; Sugars 4g; Fiber 3g; RS 1.8g; Sodium 851mg

ASK CARBLOVERS

Q: I love bread! What kinds can I eat on *CarbLovers*?

A: You can enjoy rye, pumpernickel, sourdough, and whole wheat bread on *CarbLovers*. Make sure the first ingredient listed is "whole" rye, wheat, etc., and look for 3 grams of fiber per slice.

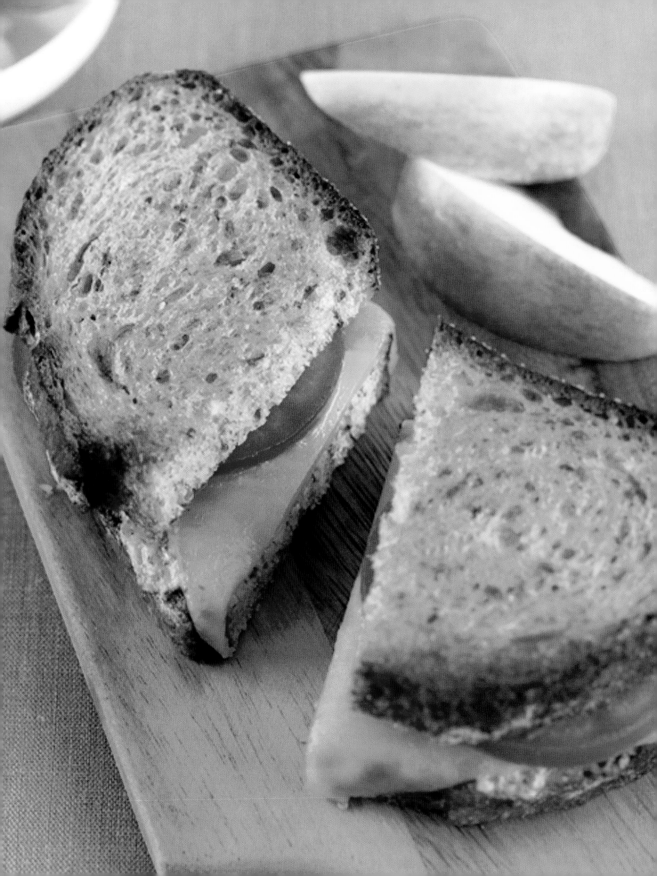

Banana-Nut Elvis Wrap

Prep: 5 minutes | *Total time:* 5 minutes | *Makes:* 4 servings

Elvis Presley was famous for eating a fried version of this sandwich. We skipped the King's melted butter and bacon and went with a whole-wheat wrap, but the PB and bananas make for a yummy combo.

½ cup chunky natural-style peanut butter
4 (6-inch) whole wheat wraps
2 large bananas, sliced
8 teaspoons honey

1. Spread 2 tablespoons peanut butter on bottom third of each wrap, leaving a 2-inch border on each side.

2. Top each wrap with ½ banana and about 2 teaspoons honey.

3. Roll up wrap, cut in half, and serve immediately.

Serving size: 1 wrap Calories 372; Fat 18.2g (sat 2.7g, mono 7.9g, poly 4.8g); Cholesterol 0mg; Protein 11g; Carbohydrate 46g; Sugars 23g; Fiber 12g; RS 3g; Sodium 247mg

Pan Bagnat

Prep: *15 minutes* | ***Total time:*** *15 minutes* | ***Makes:*** *4 servings*

This sandwich reflects the flavors of a traditional niçoise salad, and also hails from the French city of Nice. We love the briny combination of the olives, mustard, and tuna.

3 tablespoons light mayonnaise
2 tablespoons finely chopped pitted
   niçoise olives
3 teaspoons Dijon mustard
2 teaspoons red wine vinegar
½ teaspoon black pepper
1 24-inch French baguette (12
   ounces), sliced into 4 pieces,
   then halved
4 red-leaf lettuce leaves
2 medium vine-ripened tomatoes,
   sliced, each cut into 6 slices
2 hard-boiled eggs, each cut into
   6 slices
1 small red onion, cut into 8 rings
2 medium red-skinned potatoes
   (6 ounces), cooked and cooled,
   each cut into 4 slices
2 (7-ounce) jars oil-packed tuna,
   well drained

1. Whisk together mayonnaise, olives, mustard, vinegar, and pepper until smooth; chill until ready to use.

2. Spread about 2¼ teaspoons of the mayo mixture on each side of bread. Layer 1 lettuce leaf, 3 tomato slices, 3 egg slices, 2 onion rings, 2 potato slices, and about 3 ounces of tuna on bottom half of bread. Top with other bread half, slice in half on the diagonal, and serve.

Serving size: 1 sandwich Calories 507; Fat 14.1g (sat 2.9g, mono 4.8g, poly 5.2g); Cholesterol 108mg; Protein 34g; Carbohydrate 61g; Sugars 5g; Fiber 4g; RS 1.8g; Sodium 746mg

Pasta & Pizza

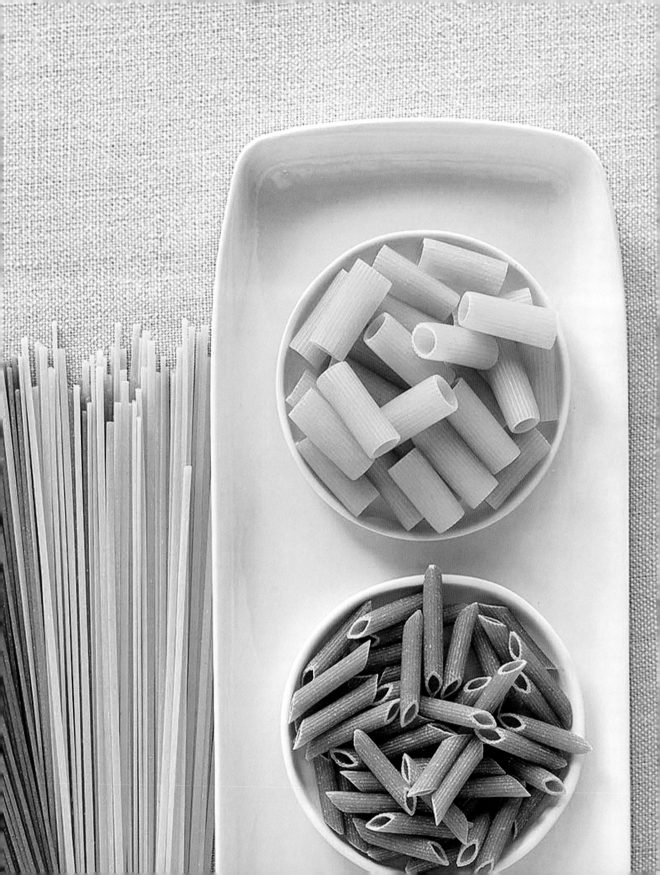

Pasta Primavera

Prep: *25 minutes* | **Cook:** *30 minutes* | **Total time:** *55 minutes* | **Makes:** *4 servings*

This delightful pasta is as gorgeous on the plate as it is delicious. We love the whimsical bow-tie shape, but feel free to substitute any pasta.

- 1 tablespoon olive oil
- 1 small onion, sliced
- 3 cloves garlic, thinly sliced
- ½ pound small multicolored cherry tomatoes
- 3 cups low-fat milk (1%)
- 3 tablespoons flour
- ½ teaspoon salt
- ½ teaspoon pepper
- 8 ounces farfalle (bow-tie) pasta
- 3 small carrots (6 ounces), peeled and diced
- ½ pound thin asparagus, trimmed and cut into 2-inch pieces
- 1 small zucchini, halved and cut into 2-inch matchsticks
- ¼ cup fresh basil leaves
- ½ cup finely shredded Parmesan cheese (½ ounce), divided

1. Bring a large pot of water to a boil.

2. While water is heating, heat oil in a large nonstick skillet over medium-high heat.

3. Add onion and cook, stirring, until soft, 6–7 minutes. Add garlic and cook 1 minute. Add tomatoes and cook (do not stir) until slightly bursting, 5 minutes.

4. Whisk together milk and flour and add to vegetables. Bring mixture to a boil; reduce heat and simmer. Stir until thickened, 2–3 minutes. Add salt and pepper, stir to incorporate, remove from heat, and cover with foil to keep warm.

5. Cook pasta according to package directions. During last 3 minutes of cooking, add carrots to boiling pasta. During last minute of cooking, add asparagus and zucchini.

6. Drain pasta and vegetables (do not rinse); add immediately to warmed vegetable-cream sauce.

7. Toss gently and divide among 4 pasta bowls.

8. Divide basil and Parmesan among bowls.

Serving size: 2 cups pasta and 2 tablespoons cheese
Calories 286; Fat 7.2g (sat 2.5g, mono 3.4g, poly 0.8g); Cholesterol 12mg; Protein 14g; Carbohydrate 43g; Sugars 15g; Fiber 5g; RS 0.6g; Sodium 473mg

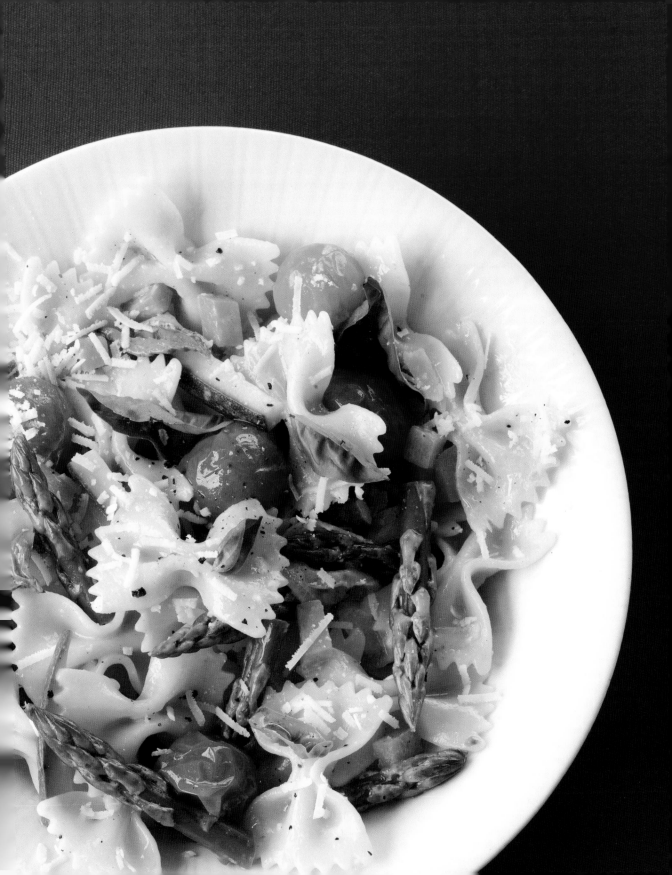

Ultimate Spinach and Turkey Lasagna

Prep: *25 minutes* | **Cook:** *1 hour 15 minutes* | **Total time:** *1 hour 40 minutes* | **Makes:** *9 servings*

*Cheesy, meaty, and unbelievably good, this saucy lasagna is a real crowd-pleaser.
Serve it with a crisp green salad.*

1	tablespoon olive oil
1	medium onion, chopped (2 cups)
2	minced garlic cloves
¾	pound ground turkey breast
3	cups low-sodium jarred marinara sauce
1½	cups part-skim ricotta cheese
1	10 ounce package frozen spinach, completely defrosted and squeezed of all excess liquid
¼	cup chopped parsley
2	egg whites
¼	teaspoon salt
¼	teaspoon pepper
12	lasagna noodles, cooked al dente according to package instructions
½	cup shredded part-skim mozzarella cheese
¼	cup shredded Parmesan cheese

1. Preheat oven to 375°.

2. Heat oil in a large high-sided skillet and cook onion, stirring occasionally, until softened, 6–7 minutes. Add garlic and cook 1 minute. Add turkey and cook, breaking up with a spoon, until no longer pink and cooked through, 4–5 minutes. Add marinara, bring to a boil, reduce heat, and simmer 2–3 minutes. Remove pan from heat and cool slightly.

3. Combine ricotta, spinach, parsley, egg whites, salt, and pepper in a large bowl.

4. Coat the bottom of a 14- x 11-inch lasagna pan with ½ cup sauce. Arrange three lasagna noodles on the bottom of the pan. Spread ¾ cup sauce evenly over noodles. Spoon ⅔ cup ricotta-spinach mixture evenly on top of sauce. Repeat layers two more times.

5. Cover top with three noodles and remaining ¾ cup sauce. Sprinkle with mozzarella and Parmesan. Cover loosely with foil and bake for 45 minutes. Remove foil and bake 10–15 minutes, until cheese is bubbly. Cut into 9 squares and serve.

Serving size: 1 (4- by 3-inch) piece Calories 346; Fat 11.3g (sat 4.3g, mono 3.7g, poly 1.5g); Cholesterol 44mg; Protein 23g; Carbohydrate 38g; Sugars 5g; Fiber 4g; RS 1g; Sodium 321mg

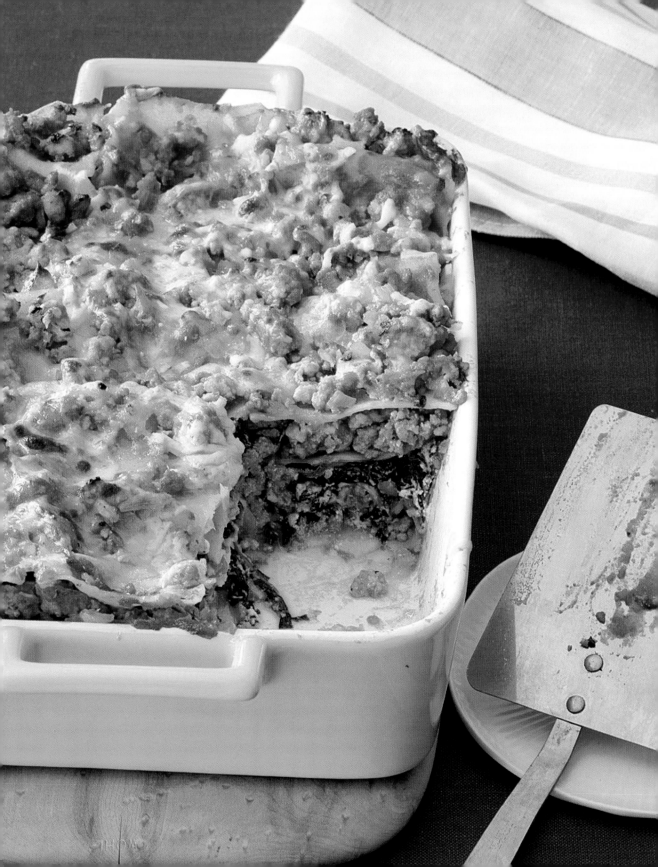

RS
2.2g

Spaghetti and Clams

Prep: 5 minutes | **Cook:** 20 minutes | **Total time**: 25 minutes | **Makes:** 4 servings

Clams have a wonderful sweet-briny flavor and add a touch of sophistication for very few calories. They're also a good source of iron.

8 ounces whole wheat spaghetti
1 tablespoon unsalted butter
1 garlic clove, thinly sliced
2 pounds littleneck or Manila
   clams, scrubbed
¼ teaspoon crushed red pepper
1 tablespoon fresh lemon juice
1 tablespoon grated Parmesan
   cheese

1. Cook spaghetti according to package directions. Reserve ½ cup of the cooking water before draining. Drain pasta and set aside.

2. Melt butter in a large skillet over medium heat. Add garlic and cook 1 minute.

3. Add clams, crushed red pepper, lemon juice, and ½ cup cooking water; stir gently to combine. Cover and simmer until clams open and release their juices, about 6 minutes. Use tongs to transfer clams to a bowl.

4. Add cooked pasta and Parmesan to the skillet with sauce. Cook, tossing, 3 minutes or until slightly thickened. Divide into 4 shallow bowls and serve.

Serving size: About 2 cups Calories 276; Fat 4.8g (sat 2.3g, mono 1g, poly 0.7g); Cholesterol 32mg; Protein 18g; Carbohydrate 44g; Sugars 1g; Fiber 4g; RS 2.2g; Sodium 208mg

TIP:
When buying fresh, live clams, make sure they are closed. Open clams should be discarded.

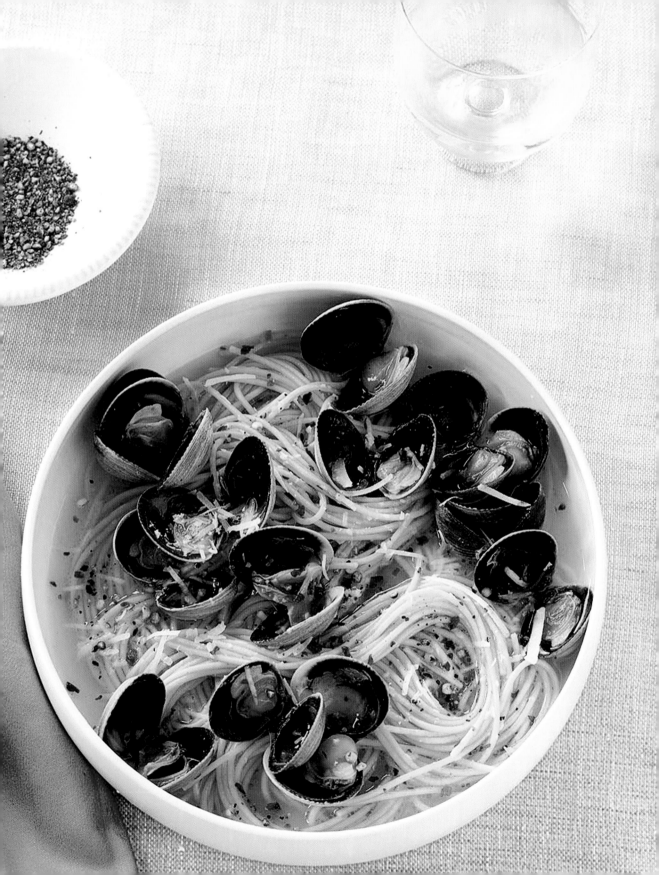

RS
1.8g

Individual Baked Mac and Cheese

Prep: *10 minutes* | **Cook:** *45 minutes* | **Total time:** *1 hour 5 minutes* | **Makes:** *6 servings*

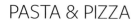

What's better than the ultimate comfort food? Your very own personal dish of it!

2½ cups low-fat milk (1%)
4 tablespoons flour
⅛ teaspoon ground or freshly grated nutmeg
3 ounces reduced-fat cheddar cheese, grated
2 ounces smoked Gouda cheese, grated
2 ounces reduced-fat Gruyère or Swiss cheese, grated
¼ teaspoon cayenne pepper
¼ teaspoon pepper
6 cups cooked elbow macaroni
1 cup unseasoned bread crumbs
2 tablespoons freshly grated Parmesan cheese
2 teaspoons chopped thyme
2 teaspoons chopped parsley
1 teaspoon olive oil or butter
¼ teaspoon salt
¼ teaspoon pepper

1. Preheat oven to 400°.

2. Whisk together milk and flour in a medium saucepan and bring to a boil over high heat. Reduce heat, add nutmeg, and cook, stirring until thickened, about 10 minutes.

3. Add cheddar, Gouda, Gruyère, cayenne, and pepper; whisk until melted, 1 minute. Add macaroni and stir to combine.

4. Toss bread crumbs, Parmesan, thyme, parsley, oil, salt, and pepper in a small bowl.

5. Place six individual crocks, ramekins, or ovenproof bowls on a rimmed baking sheet. Spoon 1 cup macaroni mixture into each ramekin and sprinkle with ⅙ cup bread-crumb topping.

6. Bake until topping is browned and cheese is bubbling, 30–35 minutes. Serve hot.

Serving size: 1 cup macaroni mixture and ⅙ cup bread-crumb topping Calories 433; Fat 12.1g (sat 6.7g, mono 1.9g, poly 0.7g); Cholesterol 34mg; Protein 22g; Carbohydrate 58g; Sugars 7g; Fiber 3g; RS 1.8g; Sodium 424mg

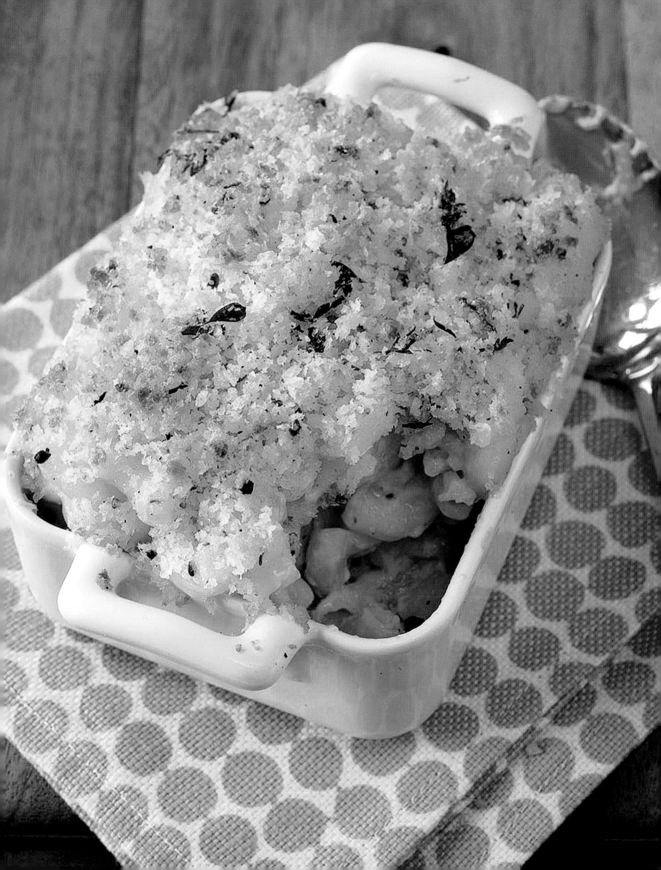

RS
5.3g

Sausage, Tomato, White Bean, and Corkscrew Pasta Toss

Prep: *5 minutes* | **Cook:** *20 minutes* | **Total time:** *25 minutes* | **Makes:** *4 servings*

Looking for a pasta meal that will keep you full for hours? This flavorful dish fits the bill with Italian sausage, beans, tomatoes—and more than 5 grams of Resistant Starch.

1 tablespoon olive oil

2 links (6 ounces) Italian sausage

1 (26-ounce) can diced tomatoes in juice

1 (15-ounce) can unsalted cannellini beans, rinsed and drained

2 teaspoons dried oregano or 1 teaspoon fresh

½ teaspoon crushed red pepper

½ pound whole wheat fusilli (corkscrew) pasta, cooked according to package directions

¼ cup freshly grated Parmesan cheese

2 tablespoons chopped parsley

1. Heat oil in a skillet over medium-high heat.

2. Add sausage and cook until browned and cooked through, 6–8 minutes. Transfer to a cutting board and thinly slice.

3. Add tomatoes with juice, beans, oregano, and crushed red pepper; bring to a low boil.

4. Reduce heat; cook until the liquid reduces slightly, about 3–4 minutes.

5. Stir in pasta; heat through, 2–3 minutes.

6. Divide among 4 bowls. Garnish each bowl with 1 tablespoon Parmesan and ½ tablespoon of the chopped parsley.

Serving size: 2¼ cups pasta Calories 435; Fat 10.1g (sat 2.9g, mono 4.6g, poly 1g); Cholesterol 17mg; Protein 24g; Carbohydrate 65g; Sugars 8g; Fiber 12g; RS 5.3g; Sodium 365mg

ASK CARBLOVERS

Q: **I'm on a budget. Can *CarbLovers* help?**

A: Absolutely! Most of the ingredients on *CarbLovers* are wallet-friendly. To save even more money, try buying grains—pasta, barley, and brown rice—in bulk. Then store them in air-tight containers away from heat and light. This will help them last a whole lot longer.

Penne with Grilled Chicken and Vodka Sauce

Prep: 10 minutes | **Cook:** 30 minutes | **Total time:** 40 minutes | **Makes:** 6 servings

This restaurant favorite is usually made with bucket-loads of heavy cream and butter. We opted to use a little olive oil and half-and-half (lighter than cream), which still gives you a wonderful, creamy texture.

1 tablespoon olive oil
1 small onion, finely diced (1 cup)
2 minced garlic cloves
1 (26-ounce) low-sodium can diced tomatoes in juice
1 (8-ounce) can no-salt-added tomato sauce
½ cup vodka
¼ teaspoon crushed red pepper
¼ cup half-and-half
¼ teaspoon salt
¼ teaspoon freshly ground pepper
4 cups cooked whole wheat penne pasta
3 (4-ounce) grilled boneless, skinless chicken breasts
2 tablespoons chopped fresh basil

1. Heat oil in a medium saucepan over medium-high heat. Add onion and cook until soft and translucent, 6–7 minutes. Add garlic and cook 1 minute.

2. Add tomatoes with juice, tomato sauce, vodka, and crushed red pepper, then bring to a boil.

5. Reduce heat and cook, stirring occasionally, until sauce reduces slightly, about 10 minutes.

6. Add half-and-half, and cook until sauce reduces, 5 minutes. Stir in salt and pepper.

8. Place ⅔ cup pasta in a bowl and top with ½ cup vodka sauce.

9. Arrange 2 ounces grilled chicken on top of pasta and garnish with chopped basil.

Serving size: ⅔ cup pasta, ½ cup sauce, and 2 ounces chicken Calories 360; Fat 6.3g (sat 1.8g, mono 2.8g, poly 1g); Cholesterol 52mg; Protein 25g; Carbohydrate 39g; Sugars 7g; Fiber 4g; RS 1g; Sodium 206mg

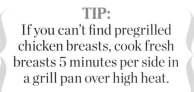

TIP:
If you can't find pregrilled chicken breasts, cook fresh breasts 5 minutes per side in a grill pan over high heat.

RS
1.5g

Chicken Cacciatore with Rigatoni

Prep: 15 minutes | *Cook:* 45 minutes | *Total time:* 1 hour | *Makes:* 4 servings

The word cacciatore *means hunter in Italian, and this hearty, rich dish is certainly fit for a hunter's appetite. We suggest choosing a glass of red wine to pair with the meal as one of your daily snacks.*

1 tablespoon olive oil
1 pound boneless, skinless chicken thighs
1 medium onion, chopped
4 sliced garlic cloves
2 cups sliced mushrooms
1 tablespoon chopped fresh oregano
1 (28-ounce) can whole tomatoes in juice, chopped
1 tablespoon tomato paste
¼ cup dry red wine
¼ teaspoon salt
¼ teaspoon black pepper
4 cups cooked rigatoni pasta
¼ cup chopped fresh parsley

1. Heat oil in a large nonstick skillet over medium-high heat. Add chicken to skillet and brown until golden, turning once, 3 minutes per side. Remove chicken from pan and reserve.

2. Reduce heat to medium; add onion and cook until soft and translucent, 6–7 minutes. Add garlic and cook 1 minute. Add mushrooms and oregano and cook until mushrooms release their water, 5 minutes.

3. Add tomatoes with juices, tomato paste, wine, salt, and pepper; simmer until slightly reduced, 5 minutes. Return chicken to skillet; spoon with some of sauce. Reduce heat to medium-low, cover, and simmer until chicken is cooked through, 20–25 minutes. Remove from heat; transfer chicken to a plate.

4. Toss pasta with sauce in a large bowl. Place 1 cup pasta with sauce in each of 4 serving bowls. Top with 2 chicken thighs, sprinkle with parsley, and serve.

Serving size: 1–2 thighs, ¾ cup sauce from pan, and 1 cup pasta Calories 462; Fat 9.6g (sat 1.9g, mono 4.1g, poly 2.1g); Cholesterol 94mg; Protein 34g; Carbohydrate 58g; Sugars 8g; Fiber 6g; RS 1.5g; Sodium 567mg

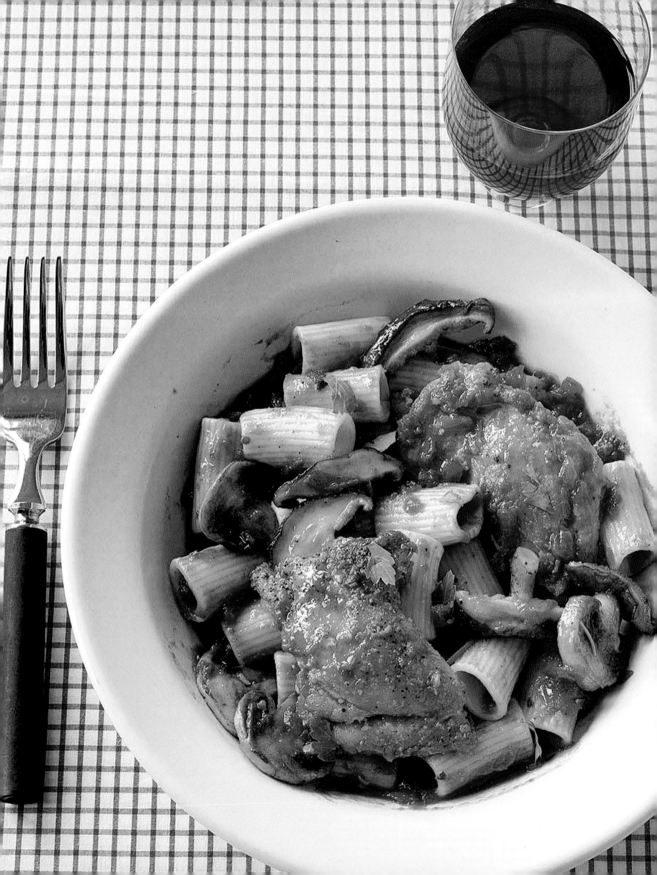

RS
1.6g

Capellini with Bacon and Bread Crumbs

Prep: *10 minutes* | **Cook:** *15 minutes* | **Total time:** *25 minutes* | **Makes:** *4 servings*

Friends coming for dinner? This quick recipe delivers restaurant-quality flavor and appeal in no time.

8   ounces whole wheat or regular capellini
2   bacon slices, chopped
1   garlic clove, sliced
¼   teaspoon crushed red pepper, optional
1   pint grape tomatoes, halved
1   cup low-sodium chicken broth
1   tablespoon olive oil
¼   cup panko bread crumbs
¼   teaspoon salt
⅛   teaspoon freshly ground black pepper
1   tablespoon freshly grated Parmesan cheese, divided
¼   cup coarsely chopped parsley

1. Cook pasta according to package directions until al dente. When pasta is done, reserve ½ cup cooking water; drain pasta and return to pot.

2. Meanwhile, heat a large skillet over medium heat; add bacon. Cook, stirring, until bacon is crispy, about 5 minutes. Add garlic and crushed red pepper; stir 1 minute or until fragrant. Add tomatoes; cook, stirring occasionally, until tomatoes begin to soften, about 3 minutes.

3. Add broth to pan. Simmer the mixture until broth is thick and has reduced to about ¼ cup, 5–8 minutes.

4. While sauce cooks, heat oil in a small skillet over medium heat. Add panko and toast, stirring occasionally, until golden, 2–3 minutes.

5. Season with salt and pepper.

6. Remove sauce from heat; stir in 2 teaspoons Parmesan and parsley.

7. Toss sauce with pasta in pot; add cooking water to reach desired consistency, if needed.

8. Divide among 4 serving plates. Top with reserved bread crumbs and remaining Parmesan.

Serving size: About 2 cups Calories 274; Fat 9.5g (sat 2.5g, mono 4.9g, poly 1.2g); Cholesterol 9mg; Protein 10g; Carbohydrate 39g; Sugars 4g; Fiber 6g; RS 1.6g; Sodium 290mg

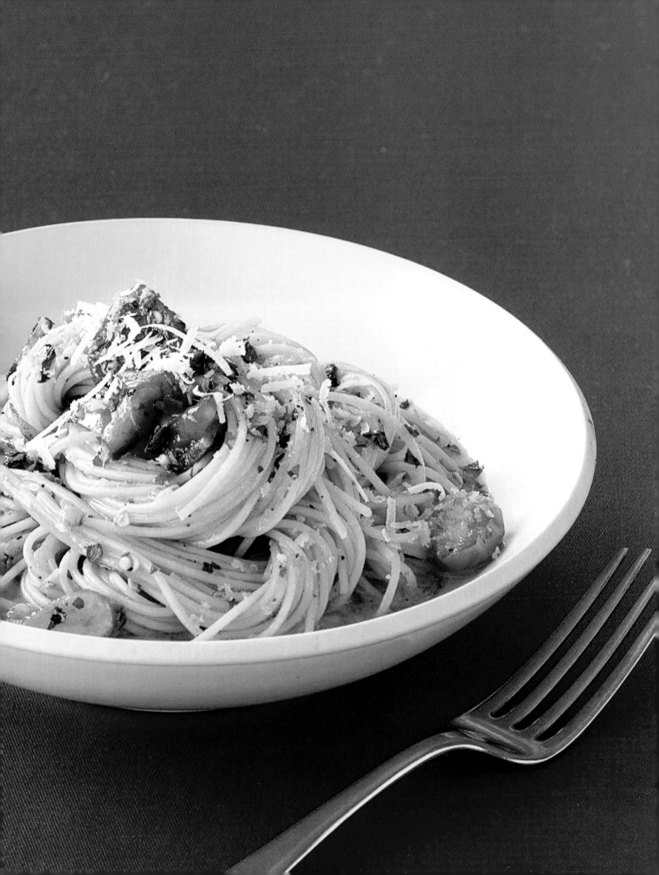

Triple-Cheese Mac

Prep: *10 minutes* | **Cook:** *20 minutes* | **Total time:** *30 minutes* | **Makes:** *6 servings*

Macaroni and cheese needn't be a diet disaster. We added high-fiber cauliflower to this version, which virtually blends into the smooth sauce. And the three cheeses provide unbelievable flavor and creaminess—yum!

1 (12-ounce) can evaporated fat-free milk
2 teaspoons Dijon mustard
⅛ teaspoon cayenne pepper
¼ teaspoon ground nutmeg
1 garlic clove, finely grated
1 (10-ounce) package frozen cauliflower florets, thawed
1 tablespoon cornstarch
1 (13.5-ounce) box whole-wheat pasta shells
½ cup coarsely grated extra-sharp cheddar cheese
½ cup coarsely grated Gouda cheese
2 tablespoons grated Parmesan cheese
2 tablespoons chopped parsley, for serving (optional)

1. Combine evaporated milk, mustard, cayenne, nutmeg, garlic, and cauliflower in a medium saucepan. Cook over medium heat, stirring occasionally, until cauliflower is tender, 5 minutes.

2. Carefully transfer to a blender; add cornstarch and blend until smooth. Return cauliflower mixture to saucepan and heat over low heat.

3. Meanwhile, cook pasta shells according to package directions. Reserve ½ cup cooking water; drain.

4. Bring sauce to a simmer until thickened; stir in cheeses. Stir until smooth. Toss sauce with pasta and, if needed, some of the cooking water. Divide into 6 bowls, top with parsley if desired, and serve immediately.

Serving size: 1¼ cups Calories 358; Fat 7.4g (sat 4.2g, mono 1.9g, poly 0.6g); Cholesterol 24mg; Protein 20g; Carbohydrate 57g; Sugars 9g; Fiber 6g; RS 2.5g; Sodium 283mg

> **TIP:**
> This cheesy dish packs ⅓ of your daily calcium needs and 2.5g of Resistant Starch, so you can feel great about digging in!

Creamy Barley Risotto with Peas and Pesto

Prep: *5 minutes* | **Cook:** *25 minutes* | **Total time:** *30 minutes* | **Makes:** *4 servings*

Once you try this dish, you'll be a convert to barley. Its wonderful nutty flavor and slightly chewy texture make it a star in creamy dishes, as well as in cold salads.

1 tablespoon olive oil
1 shallot, finely chopped
2 garlic cloves, finely chopped
2 cups pearl barley
2 cups reduced-sodium chicken broth
½ teaspoon salt
¼ teaspoon freshly ground black pepper
1 cup frozen peas, thawed
2 tablespoons finely grated Parmesan cheese
3 tablespoons store-bought pesto, for serving

1. Heat oil in a medium skillet over medium-high heat. Add shallot and garlic; cook 4–5 minutes until onion begins to brown.

2. Reduce heat to medium; stir in barley and broth. Cook, stirring occasionally, until liquid is absorbed, about 10 minutes. Add 2 cups water; cook until vegetables are tender and most of the liquid has been absorbed, 10–15 minutes. Season with salt and pepper.

3. Stir in peas; remove from heat. Let risotto rest 1–2 minutes until peas are thawed but still bright green. Stir in Parmesan just before serving. Serve topped with pesto.

Serving size: 1⅛ cups Calories 423; Fat 10.5g (sat 2.1g, mono 2.8g, poly 0.9g); Cholesterol 6mg; Protein 10g; Carbohydrate 74g; Sugars 3g; Fiber 11g; RS 6.5g; Sodium 637mg

Gnocchi with Walnut-Arugula Pesto

Prep: *5 minutes* | **Cook:** *5 minutes* | **Total time:** *10 minutes* | **Makes:** *4 servings*

These little Italian potato dumplings make for a delicious, filling, and superfast meal.

6   cups loosely packed arugula, divided
1¼ cups (1½ ounces) freshly grated Parmesan cheese, divided
¼   cup walnuts
½   teaspoon salt
¼   teaspoon freshly ground black pepper
2   tablespoons olive oil
1   (14-ounce) package frozen, store-bought potato gnocchi

1. Place 4 cups arugula, 1 cup Parmesan, walnuts, salt, and pepper in a food processor; pulse until incorporated, 30 seconds. With motor running, drizzle in oil and 1 tablespoon water; process until smooth, 30 seconds, adding more water by the tablespoon if necessary.

2. Cook gnocchi according to package directions; drain. Return gnocchi to pot; add pesto.

3. Divide remaining arugula among 4 bowls; toss with the gnocchi. Sprinkle with remaining Parmesan, and serve immediately.

Serving size: 2 cups gnocchi-arugula mixture
Calories 358; Fat 25.1g (sat 9.9g, mono 9.6g, poly 4.4g); Cholesterol 41mg; Protein 14g; Carbohydrate 21g; Sugars 1g; Fiber 2g; RS 1.6g; Sodium 605mg

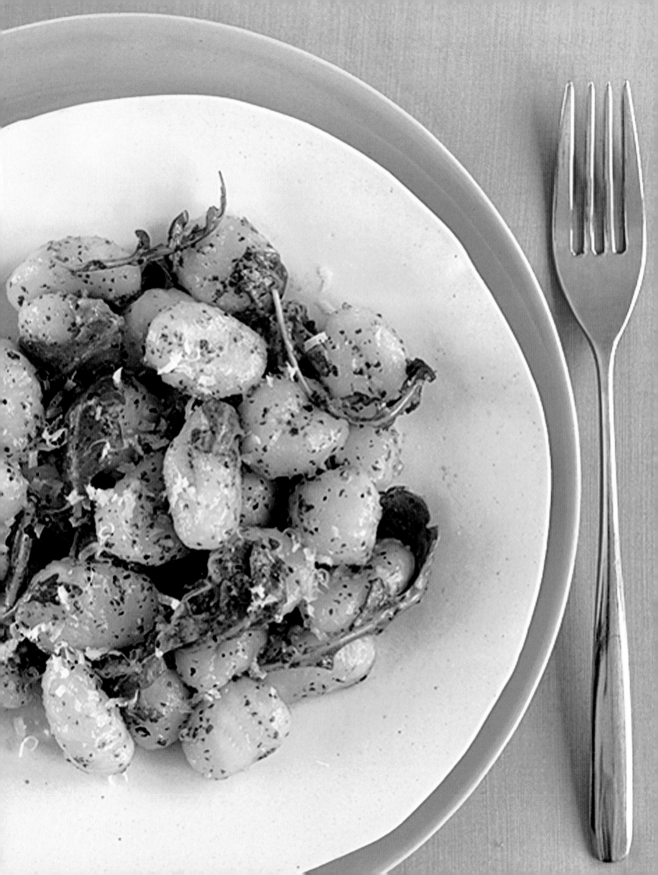

Spaghetti and Turkey Meatballs in Tomato Sauce

Prep: *15 minutes* | **Cook:** *30 minutes* | **Total time:** *45 minutes* | **Makes:** *5 servings*

The whole family will love this yummy and ultra-satisfying dish. We took classic spaghetti and meatballs and made it healthier by using lean turkey and adding beans to boost the Resistant Starch. The end result is as delicious as you'd expect!

1 pound ground lean turkey meat
¾ cup finely grated Parmesan cheese, divided
¼ cup chopped parsley, plus more for garnish
¼ cup fresh whole wheat bread crumbs (from 1 slice bread)
1 egg, beaten
¾ teaspoon salt, divided
½ teaspoon pepper, divided
1 tablespoon olive oil
1 small onion, minced (1 cup)
2 minced garlic cloves
1 (26-ounce) can low-sodium crushed tomatoes
1 cup canned pinto beans, rinsed and drained
½ pound whole wheat spaghetti, cooked according to package directions and kept warm

1. Combine turkey, ½ cup Parmesan, parsley, bread crumbs, egg, ½ teaspoon salt, and ¼ teaspoon pepper in a bowl; form into 15 meatballs. Place meatballs on a plate and set aside.

2. Heat oil in a large saucepan over medium-high heat. Add onion; cook until soft, 5 minutes. Add garlic; cook 2 minutes.

3. Add tomatoes, beans, and remaining salt and pepper; bring to a boil.

4. Add meatballs; return to a boil. Reduce heat and simmer over low heat until meatballs are cooked through and sauce has thickened, 15 minutes.

5. Divide spaghetti among 5 bowls, then divide meatballs and sauce among bowls. Garnish with additional parsley and remaining ¼ cup Parmesan.

Serving size: 1 cup pasta, 3 meatballs, and about ¾ cup sauce Calories 439; Fat 12.2g (sat 3.4g, mono 2.7g, poly 1g); Cholesterol 98mg; Protein 33g; Carbohydrate 55g; Sugars 2g; Fiber 9g; RS 2.5g; Sodium 623mg

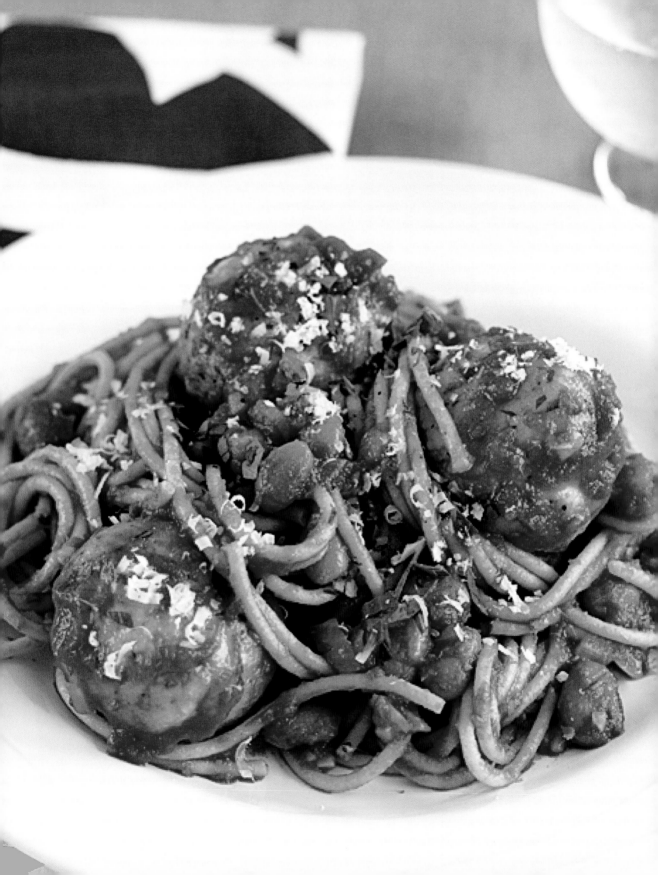

RS
3.5g

Pasta with Peas, Ham, and Parmesan Cheese

Prep: 5 minutes | **Cook:** 15 minutes | **Total time:** 20 minutes | **Makes:** 4 servings

We tossed bow ties, sweet peas, and salty ham in a creamy sauce to create a really rich-tasting, but still light dish you will absolutely love.

½ cup light sour cream
1 (10-ounce) box frozen peas, thawed
8 ounces uncooked whole-wheat orecchiette or bow-tie pasta
4 ounces lean, boneless ham, thinly sliced
1 cup finely grated Parmesan cheese, divided
2 tablespoons chopped fresh tarragon, plus more for garnish
½ teaspoon salt
½ teaspoon pepper

1. Combine sour cream and peas in a small bowl.

2. Cook pasta according to package directions. Drain, reserving ¼ cup of the cooking water.

3. Return pasta to pot. Fold in sour cream mixture, ham, ¾ cup Parmesan, tarragon, salt, and pepper. Stir in enough reserved cooking water to create a thin sauce.

4. Divide among 4 bowls; garnish with additional tarragon and remaining Parmesan.

Serving size: 2 cups pasta Calories 434; Fat 12.7g (sat 6.6g, mono 4g, poly 1g); Cholesterol 55mg; Protein 29g; Carbohydrate 54g; Sugars 5g; Fiber 8g; RS 3.5g; Sodium 538mg

ASK CARBLOVERS

Q: **I haven't really eaten pasta in years. How can I make friends with this food again?**

A: Pasta should be enjoyed in modest portions with fresh herbs, vegetables, lean meats, interesting sauces, and even nuts and beans. Experiment!

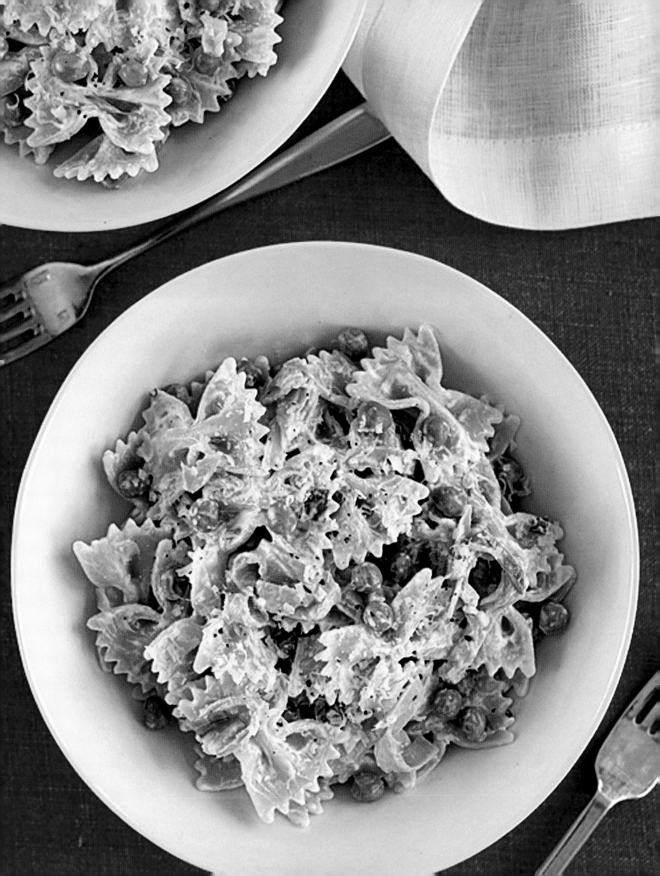

RS
3.3g

Penne with Sausage and Spinach

Prep: 5 minutes | **Cook:** 20 minutes | **Total time:** 25 minutes | **Makes:** 4 servings

It's tough to find dishes that are satisfying both to your taste buds and to your health standards, but this one delivers both. You get to indulge in savory sausage and pasta while getting 8 grams of fiber and more than 3 grams of Resistant Starch.

12 ounces whole wheat penne
 1 tablespoon olive oil
 3 Italian turkey sausages
 1 cup reduced-sodium chicken broth
¼ teaspoon crushed red pepper (optional)
 1 (5-ounce) container baby spinach
 2 tablespoons grated Pecorino cheese
 1 tablespoon fresh lemon juice

1. Cook pasta according to package directions.

2. Meanwhile, heat oil in a large skillet over medium-high heat. Remove sausage from casing; form each link into 4 balls.

3. Add meatballs to skillet; cook, tossing occasionally, until browned, about 5 minutes. Add broth and, if using, crushed red pepper; simmer 8 minutes or until broth is almost fully evaporated.

4. Add the cooked pasta to the skillet, then stir in spinach to wilt.

5. Toss pasta and spinach with Pecorino and lemon juice. Transfer to 4 bowls and serve while hot.

Serving size: 2½ cups Calories 447; Fat 11g (sat 3g, mono 2.6g, poly 0.9g); Cholesterol 56mg; Protein 26g; Carbohydrate 66g; Sugars 2g; Fiber 8g; RS 3.3g; Sodium 600mg

Roasted Eggplant and Ricotta Calzones

Prep: *20 minutes* | ***Cook:*** *35 minutes* | ***Total time:*** *55 minutes* | ***Makes:*** *6 servings*

Filled with lots of rich cheese and pepperoni, calzones generally aren't considered diet fare. We slimmed ours down by using part-skim ricotta and swapping sausage for roasted eggplant, which adds a ton of flavor and fiber with very few calories.

1 medium (1 pound) eggplant, cubed (about 5 cups)
2 tablespoons olive oil
½ teaspoon pepper, divided
3 cups jarred marinara sauce, divided
1 cup part-skim ricotta cheese
2 tablespoons chopped parsley
½ cup chopped fresh basil
¼ cup cornmeal, divided
1 whole wheat pizza dough (1 pound), divided into 6 equal-size pieces
1 egg white, beaten

1. Preheat oven to 500°.

2. Toss eggplant with oil and ¼ teaspoon pepper. Place in a single layer on a foil-lined baking sheet; bake until soft and edges are charred, 15 minutes. Remove eggplant from oven and cool to room temperature.

3. Transfer cooked eggplant to a bowl and toss with 2 cups marinara.

4. Combine ricotta, parsley, basil, and remaining pepper in a small bowl until incorporated.

5. Sprinkle 2 tablespoons cornmeal on a clean, dry work surface. Place one dough ball on surface and roll out to a 9-inch circle. Place about ¾ cup eggplant filling and about ¼ cup ricotta mixture in center of circle. Moisten edges with water, fold into a half moon, and crimp tightly with fingers to close. Repeat with remaining pieces of dough.

6. Transfer calzones to a parchment-lined baking sheet and brush with egg white. Bake until golden brown, 16–17 minutes.

7. Serve with additional warmed marinara sauce for dipping.

Serving size: 1 calzone and about 2½ tablespoons sauce
Calories 380; Fat 12.9g (sat 2.7g, mono 4.3g, poly 0.7g); Cholesterol 13mg; Protein 14g; Carbohydrate 53g; Sugars 6g; Fiber 7g; RS 5.3g; Sodium 798mg

RS
2.2g

Fresh Mozzarella, Basil, and Chicken Sausage Pizza

Prep: 5 minutes | **Cook:** 20 minutes | **Total time:** 25 minutes | **Makes:** 6 servings

Delicious mozzarella: check. Sausage: check. Spicy tomato sauce: check. Resistant Starch: check! Finally, even dieters can have an amazing, pizzeria-style pie at home.

1   pound fresh or frozen whole wheat pizza dough, thawed
1   tablespoon olive oil
2   medium tomatoes (about 10 ounces)
¼   teaspoon crushed red pepper
¼   teaspoon dried oregano
½   cup fresh basil leaves, divided
8   ounces fresh mozzarella, pulled into 1-inch chunks
2   links (6 ounces total) precooked Italian chicken sausage (such as Applegate brand), sliced

1. Position one oven rack in middle of oven and another on the lowest setting. Place a flat baking sheet on the bottom rack. Preheat oven to 475°.

2. Roll dough into a large, thin oval (about 18 inches long). Brush oil over dough.

3. Remove preheated baking sheet from oven. Slide dough onto sheet and return to bottom rack. Bake for 8 minutes, then remove crust from oven.

4. Meanwhile, with clean hands, crush tomatoes, crushed red pepper, oregano, and ¼ cup basil in a medium bowl.

5. Spread sauce in an even layer over crust, leaving a ¼-inch border. Top with mozzarella and sausage. Bake on middle rack an additional 10 minutes or until crust is golden brown and cheese melts. Sprinkle with remaining basil; cut into 12 slices or wedges and serve.

Serving size: 2 slices pizza Calories 360; Fat 17.9g (sat 7.4g, mono 2.4g, poly 0.7g); Cholesterol 51mg; Protein 17.2g; Carbohydrate 32g; Sugars 1g; Fiber 3g; RS 2.2g; Sodium 322mg

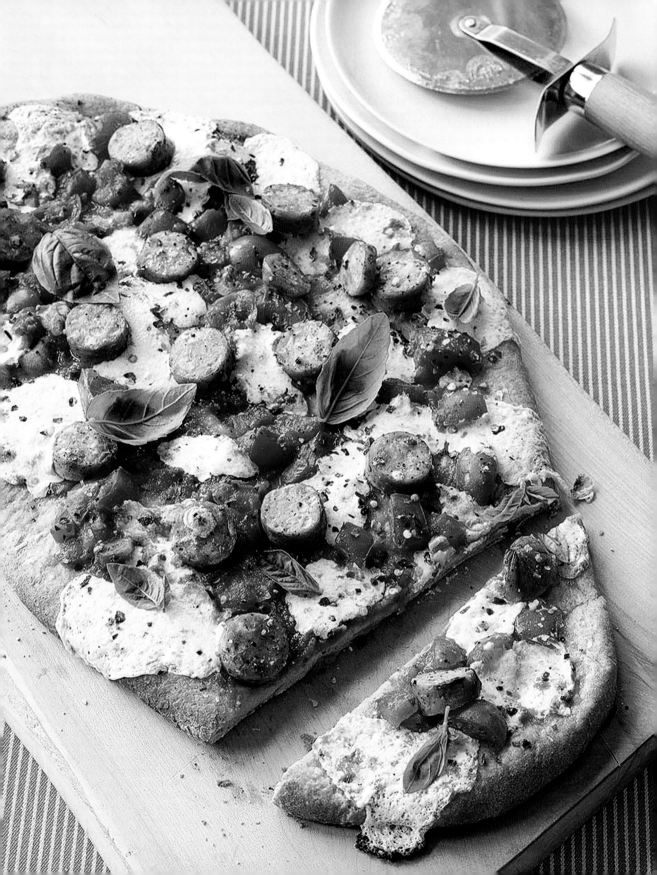

RS
2g

Pizza with Prosciutto, Tomatoes, and Parmesan Cheese

Prep: 5 minutes | **Cook:** 15 minutes | **Total time:** 20 minutes | **Makes:** 4 servings

Dinner in 20 is easy to pull off with this tempting pizza. Serve it with a fresh green salad dressed with olive oil and balsamic vinegar.

1   (12-inch) prebaked whole wheat pizza crust
¾   cup low-sodium marinara sauce
½   cup shredded, part-skim mozzarella cheese
¼   cup freshly grated Parmesan cheese
2   thin slices (1 ounce) prosciutto, coarsely chopped
3   small tomatoes, sliced (4 ounces)
8   fresh basil leaves

1. Preheat oven to 400°.

2. Place pizza crust on a baking sheet.

3. Spread sauce evenly over crust, leaving a 1-inch border around the edges.

4. Combine cheeses, and sprinkle evenly over sauce. Top with prosciutto and tomatoes.

5. Bake until cheese is bubbly and crust is browned around the edges, 12–15 minutes. Remove from oven, and distribute basil leaves evenly over pizza. Let pizza rest for 5 minutes. Cut into 8 slices, and serve immediately.

Serving size: 2 slices Calories 286; Fat 9.3g (sat 3.4g, mono 1.1g, poly 0.2g); Cholesterol 18mg; Protein 17g; Carbohydrate 38g; Sugars 5g; Fiber 6g; RS 2g; Sodium 699mg

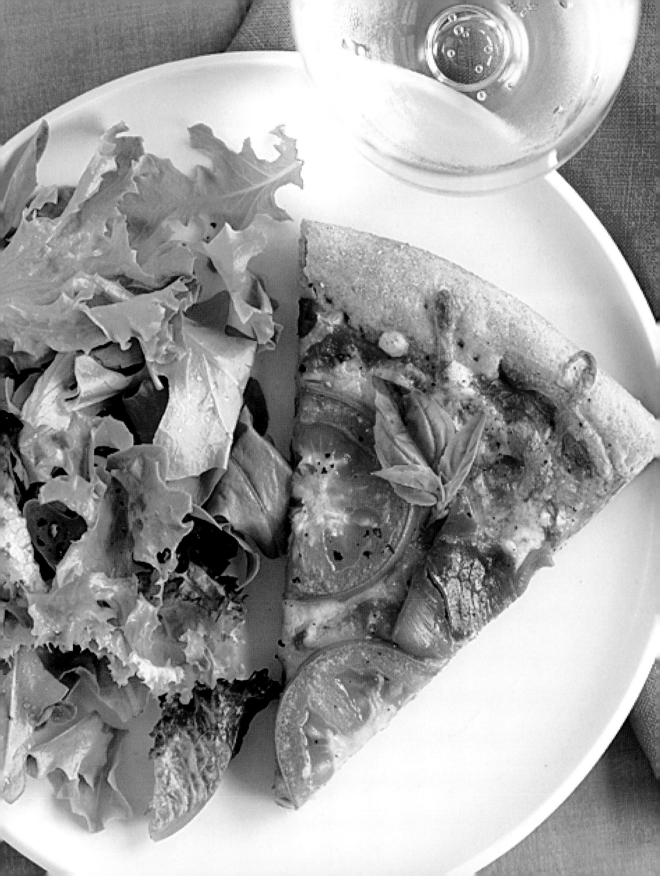

Mini Mediterranean Pizzas

Prep: *10 minutes* | **Cook:** *10 minutes* | **Total time:** *20 minutes* | **Makes:** *4 servings*

A quick lunch or dinner is just 20 minutes away with these delicious mini pizzas.

1 cup grape tomatoes
1 garlic clove, sliced
¼ teaspoon freshly ground black pepper
4 (6-inch) whole-wheat pitas
1 tablespoon olive oil, plus more for drizzling
½ cup crumbled feta cheese
¼ cup halved, pitted kalamata olives
¼ cup roasted bell peppers, sliced
1 cup baby arugula

1. Preheat oven to 450°.

2. Crush tomatoes with garlic and pepper in a small bowl.

3. Arrange 4 pitas on a large rimmed baking sheet; brush both sides of pita with oil. Top pitas with equal amounts of the tomato mixture, feta, olives, and bell peppers.

4. Bake 7–8 minutes or until edges are golden.

5. Remove pitas from oven; top each with ¼ cup arugula.

6. Drizzle with additional oil, if desired. Serve.

Serving size: 1 pizza Calories 274; Fat 8.9g (sat 3.5g, mono 4.5g, poly 0.7g); Cholesterol 17mg; Protein 10g; Carbohydrate 29g; Sugars 5g; Fiber 1g; RS 1g; Sodium 608mg

TIP:
If you aren't a fan of arugula, you can top the pizzas with baby spinach or other favorite ingredients.

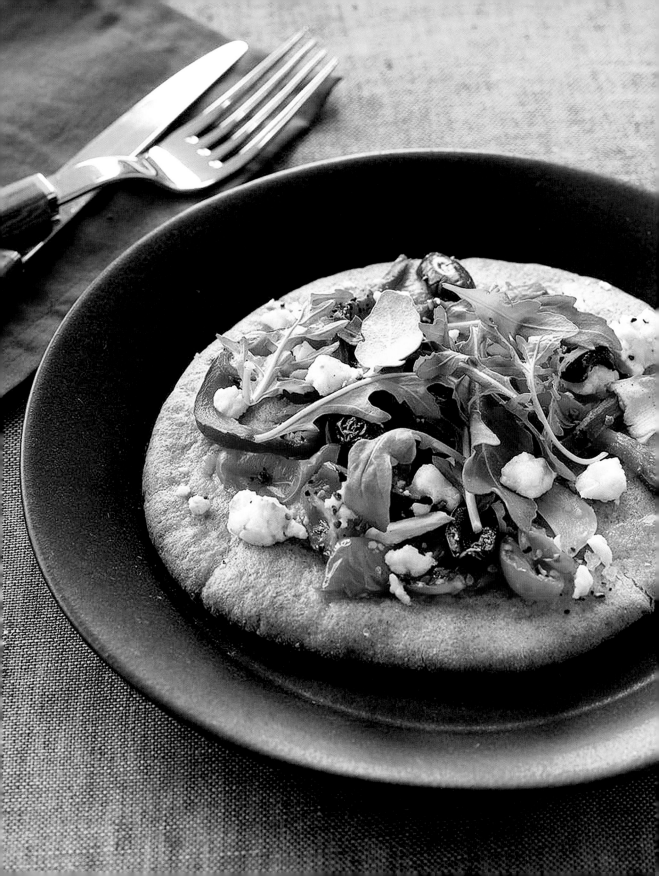

Seafood, Meat & Poultry

Maple-Glazed Cod with Baby Bok Choy

Prep: *5 minutes* | ***Cook:*** *10 minutes* | ***Total time:*** *15 minutes* | ***Makes:*** *4 servings*

Meaty and slightly sweet, heart-healthy cod lends itself to Asian-inspired dishes like this one. Serve it with brown rice for a complete meal and added Resistant Starch.

2	tablespoons maple syrup
1	tablespoon low-sodium soy sauce
1	teaspoon sesame oil
¼	teaspoon crushed red pepper
4	6 ounces skinless cod fillets
1	tablespoon canola oil
3	cloves minced garlic
1	tablespoon chopped fresh ginger
6	heads baby bok choy, halved (about 8 cups)
2	tablespoons mirin
1	tablespoon low-sodium soy sauce
1	tablespoon rice wine vinegar
4	teaspoons chopped scallions
2	teaspoons lightly toasted sesame seeds

1. Make cod: Combine maple syrup, soy sauce, sesame oil and crushed red pepper. Place fish in a glass baking dish and pour marinade over fish; refrigerate for 30 minutes or up to 2 hours.

2. Preheat oven to 475°. Transfer fillets to a foil-lined baking sheet and roast until fish is cooked through and slightly browned, 9–10 minutes.

3. Meanwhile, make bok choy: Heat canola oil in a very large skillet over medium-high heat. Add garlic and ginger and cook, stirring, until fragrant but not browned, 1 minute. Add bok choy, then follow immediately with mirin, soy sauce, and vinegar. Cook, stirring, until greens are wilted and stalks are tender-crisp, 3–4 minutes.

4. Remove fish from oven. Sprinkle each fillet with 1 teaspoon chopped scallion and ½ teaspoon toasted sesame seeds. Serve with bok choy.

Serving size: 6 ounces cod and 1 cup bok choy Calories 256; Fat 7.1g (sat 0.8g, mono 3.3g, poly 2.5g); Cholesterol 65mg; Protein 31g; Carbohydrate 16g; Sugars 11g; Fiber 3g; RS 0g; Sodium 509mg

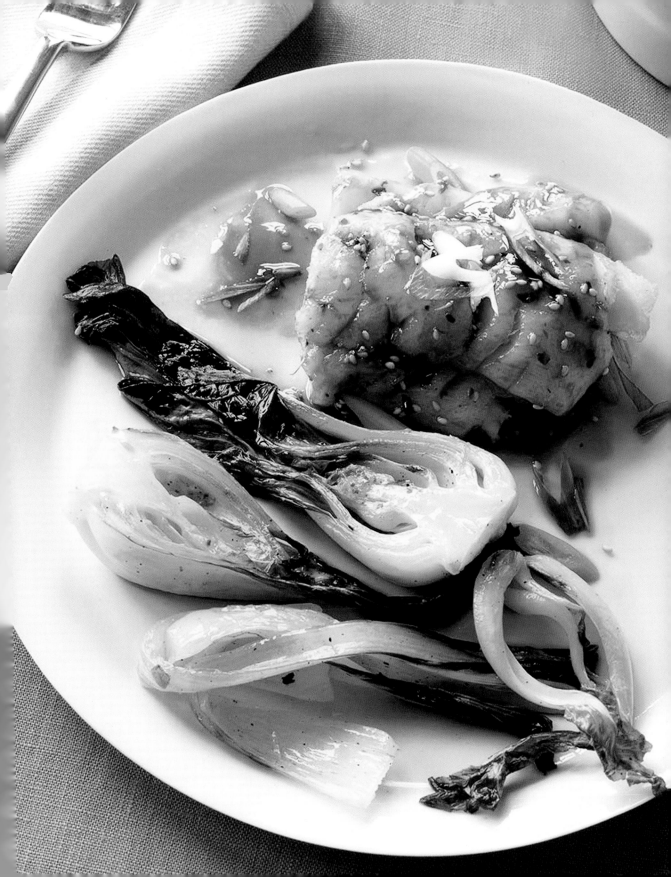

RS
2.1g

Cornmeal-Crusted Tilapia with Sautéed Greens and Whipped Honey Yams

Prep: *20 minutes* | **Cook:** *45 minutes* | **Total time:** *1 hour 5 minutes* | **Makes:** *4 servings*

This complete meal is Southern food at its finest—and skinniest!

2 pounds garnet yams, peeled and cut into 2-inch chunks
1 cup vegetable or chicken broth, divided
1 tablespoon honey
  Cooking spray
2 tablespoons vegetable oil, divided
1 small onion, chopped
3 garlic cloves, sliced
1 pound collard greens, greens separated from stems, then sliced, stems chopped
¾ teaspoon smoked paprika, divided
¼ teaspoon crushed red pepper
¼ teaspoon salt, divided
½ teaspooon pepper, divided
1 egg white, beaten
¼ cup cornmeal
4 6-ounce tilapia fillets
¼ cup flour

1. Place yams and ½ cup broth in a saucepan; bring to a boil. Reduce heat, cover, and cook until yams are fork-tender, about 20 minutes. Remove from heat, transfer to a bowl, and add honey.

2. Whip yams with a hand mixer, 2 minutes. Cover to keep warm.

3. Add 2 teaspoons oil to a large nonstick skillet coated with cooking spray; heat over medium-high heat. Add onion and cook, stirring, until lightly browned, 7–8 minutes. Add garlic, collard stems, remaining ½ cup stock, ½ teaspoon paprika, crushed red pepper, and half of the salt and pepper; cook until stems are slightly softened, 2–3 minutes. Add collard greens and cook 1–2 minutes until wilted. Remove from heat and cover with foil.

4. Place egg white in a shallow dish. Combine cornmeal and remaining salt and pepper in another shallow dish. Combine flour and remaining ¼ teaspoon paprika in a plastic bag. Dredge fish in flour, then moisten with egg white. Press into cornmeal mixture on both sides. Heat 2 teaspoons oil in a nonstick skillet over medium-high heat. Place 2 fish fillets in pan and cook until browned, 3 minutes. Flip fish and cook until cooked through, 3–4 minutes more. Repeat with remaining oil and fish.

Serving size: 1 piece fish, ¾ cup yams and 1 cup sautéed greens Calories 502; Fat 12.2g (sat 2.3g, mono 2g, poly 5g); Cholesterol 114mg; Protein 41g; Carbohydrate 60g; Sugars 17g; Fiber 10g; RS 2.1g; Sodium 513mg

RS
0.3g

Honey and Sesame–Glazed Salmon with Confetti Barley Salad

Prep: 10 minutes | *Cook:* 30 minutes | *Total time:* 40 minutes | *Makes:* 4 servings

This is truly a power meal! Omega-3-packed salmon helps boost your metabolism. And the barley kicks in Resistant Starch and fiber.

¾ cup pearl barley
1 (16-ounce) bag frozen stir-fry vegetables, thawed and chopped
1 tablespoon toasted sesame seeds, divided
4 (4-ounce) skinless salmon fillets
3 tablespoons honey
¼ cup low-sodium soy sauce
1½ teaspoon toasted sesame oil
¼ teaspoon crushed red pepper
¼ cup chopped scallions

1. Preheat oven to 400°.

2. Bring a large pot of salted water to a boil.

3. Add barley, return to a boil, and boil until tender, 30 minutes. Add vegetables during last 3 minutes of cooking. Drain, cool slightly, and toss with 2 teaspoons sesame seeds; set aside.

4. While barley is cooking, make salmon: Combine honey, soy sauce, sesame oil, and chili flakes. Reserve 4 tablespoons of mixture. Place salmon on a baking sheet, and brush with honey-soy mixture. Bake until salmon is flaky, 15 minutes. Place reserved sauce in a small saucepan over low heat, and keep warm.

5. Divide barley mixture among 4 plates, top with 1 salmon fillet and 1 tablespoon warmed sauce, and sprinkle with scallions and remaining sesame seeds.

Serving size: 1 cup barley-vegetable mixture, 4 ounces salmon, and 1 tablespoon additional sauce Calories 435; Fat 6.8g (sat 0.5g, mono 2.2g, poly 2.9g); Cholesterol 72mg; Protein 33g; Carbohydrate 53g; Sugars 16g; Fiber 9g; RS 0.3g; Sodium 615mg

RS
1.5g

Shrimp Tacos with Lime Crema

Prep: 10 minutes | **Cook:** 5 minutes | **Total:** 15 minutes | **Makes:** 4 servings

Tacos de camarones (shrimp tacos) originated in Baja California in Mexico. We love them because they're outrageously good—and take less than 20 minutes to make.

- 1 pound medium shrimp, peeled and deveined
- ¼ teaspoon chili powder
- ¼ teaspoon cumin
- ⅛ teaspoon black pepper
- 1 teaspoon olive oil
- 2 tablespoons lime juice, divided
- ½ cup reduced-fat sour cream
- 8 (6-inch) corn tortillas, warmed according to package directions
- ¼ cup finely diced red onion, for serving
- 2 cups shredded lettuce, for serving

1. Toss shrimp with chili powder, cumin, and pepper in a medium bowl. Heat oil in a large nonstick skillet over medium heat. Add shrimp; sauté 3 minutes, turning once, or until done. Remove from heat. Season with 1 tablespoon lime juice.

2. Stir together sour cream and remaining lime juice in a small bowl. To serve, fill tortillas with lettuce, top with shrimp mixture and red onion, and drizzle with lime crema.

Serving size: 2 tortillas, 2 tablespoons onion, ½ cup lettuce, 4 ounces shrimp, 2 tablespoons crema   Calories 258; Fat 7.3g (sat 2.7g, mono 2.3g, poly 1g); Cholesterol 155mg; Protein 20g; Carbohydrate 29g; Sugars 1g; Fiber 4g; RS 1.5g; Sodium 665mg

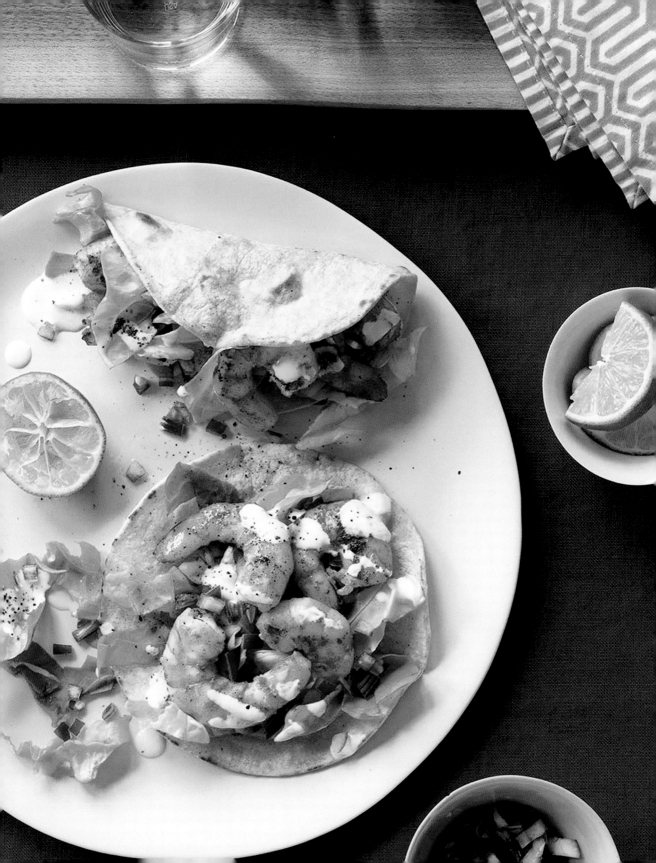

Seared Scallops with Asian Slaw

Prep: 10 minutes | *Cook:* 5 minutes | *Total time:* 15 minutes | *Makes:* 4 servings

Superlight and very quick cooking, scallops are a busy dieter's dream. We love the combination of the tangy slaw and the sweet, meaty scallops.

- 1 tablespoon finely grated ginger
- 2 tablespoons rice wine vinegar
- 1 teaspoon fish sauce (optional)
- 1½ teaspoons sugar
- 4 baby bok choy, thinly sliced (about 4 cups)
- 2 scallions, thinly sliced
- 1 teaspoon black or white sesame seeds
- 1 pound dry sea scallops (about 16)
- ¼ teaspoon kosher salt
- ¼ teaspoon freshly ground black pepper
- 2 cups cooked brown rice

1. Whisk together ginger, vinegar, fish sauce (if using), and sugar in a medium bowl. Toss with bok choy, scallions, and sesame seeds. Set aside.

2. Season scallops with salt and pepper. Heat a large nonstick skillet over medium-high heat. Place 1 scallop in center of pan. When scallop sizzles, arrange remaining scallops in pan, flat sides down (make sure they aren't touching or they will steam and not sear properly). Cook 2–3 minutes on each side until lightly browned and opaque in the center. Place ¼ of the slaw on each of 4 plates. Add ½ cup cooked brown rice and top with 4 scallops each. Serve immediately.

Serving size: 1 cup slaw, ½ cup rice, and 4 scallops
Calories 217; Fat 1.9g (sat 0.4g, mono 0.6g, poly 0.7g); Cholesterol 27mg; Protein 18g; Carbohydrate 32g; Sugars 4g; Fiber 4g; RS 1.7g; Sodium 625mg

Grilled Spice-Rubbed Pork Tenderloin with Broccoli Rabe

Prep: *10 minutes* | **Cook:** *25 Minutes* | **Total time:** *35 minutes* | **Makes:** *4 servings*

The delicious bite of broccoli rabe pairs well with the mild flavor of pork tenderloin. And the spice rub is absolutely delicious.

4 teaspoons olive oil, divided
¼ teaspoon salt, divided
1 teaspoon smoked paprika
1 teaspoon oregano
½ teaspoon pepper
1 teaspoon cumin
½ teaspoon sugar
1¼ pounds pork tenderloin
3 thinly sliced garlic cloves
1½ pounds broccoli rabe (including leaves and stalks), trimmed, stalks chopped (about 12 cups raw)

1. Combine 2 teaspoons oil, ¼ teaspoon salt and next 5 ingredients (through sugar) in a small bowl. Pat tenderloin dry and rub with spice mixture.

2. Preheat a grill or grill pan over medium-high heat. Grill tenderloin until a thermometer inserted into the thickest part of the roast reads 155°, about 8 minutes per side. Remove from heat and let rest.

3. While meat is resting, heat remaining oil over medium heat in a very large skillet. Add garlic and cook until softened and slightly browned, 2 minutes. In 2 batches add broccoli rabe and cook until crisp-tender, 3–4 minutes total, adding water by the tablespoon if the pan gets dry. Remove from heat. Slice meat against grain. Divide pork and broccoli rabe among 4 plates.

Serving size: 4 ounces pork and ¾ cup broccoli rabe
Calories 244; Fat 9.8g (sat 2.2g, mono 5g, poly 1.4g); Cholesterol 78mg; Protein 33g; Carbohydrate 7g; Sugars 1g; Fiber 5g; RS 0g; Sodium 409mg

Bison Sliders with Guacamole

Prep: 20 minutes | **Cook:** 5 minutes | **Total time:** 25 minutes | **Makes:** 4 servings

These juicy sliders are addictive! Make them for a party or an easy weeknight dinner.

1 large avocado
1 tablespoon reduced-fat sour cream
Juice and zest of 1 lime
1 tablespoon finely chopped jalapeño pepper
2 tablespoons chopped cilantro
¾ teaspoon salt, divided
½ teaspoon pepper, divided
1 pound ground bison
1 minced garlic clove
1 small head butter lettuce, inner leaves separated
2 plum tomatoes, thinly sliced
½ small red onion, sliced into rings
8 whole wheat slider buns

1. Mash avocado, sour cream, lime juice and zest, jalapeño, cilantro, ½ teaspoon salt, and ¼ teaspoon pepper in a medium bowl until chunky. Press plastic wrap onto surface of guacamole, and refrigerate.

2. Combine bison, garlic, and remaining salt and pepper in a small bowl. Form into eight 2-ounce patties, transfer to a plate, and set aside.

3. Preheat a grill or grill pan over medium-high heat. Grill sliders until thoroughly cooked; 4 minutes per side for medium.

4. Layer one lettuce leaf, a slice of tomato, and an onion ring on bottom half of each bun, and top with 2 tablespoons guacamole. Add a slider, and top with other half of bun.

Serving size: 2 sliders   Calories 444; Fat 24.2g (sat 7.6g, mono 11g, poly 2.9g); Cholesterol 61mg; Protein 23g; Carbohydrate 38g; Sugars 7g; Fiber 9g; RS 0.2g; Sodium 544mg

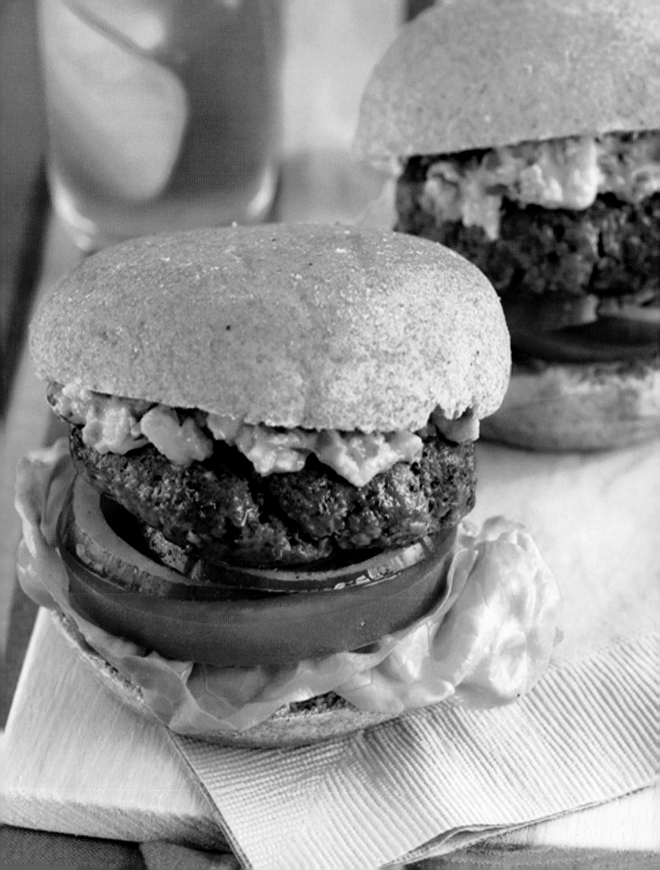

RS 2.9g

Grilled Flank Steak Fajitas

Prep: *15 minutes* | ***Cook:*** *30 minutes* | ***Total time:*** *45 minutes* | ***Makes:*** *4 servings*

Fajitas make a perfectly balanced meal. You get vegetables, lean meat, beans, and Resistant Starch–packed tortillas. Plus they're incredibly fun to eat!

¼ cup fresh lime juice plus
   2 teaspoons lime zest
¼ cup chopped cilantro
2 cloves minced garlic
2 teaspoons minced jalapeño chile
1 pound flank steak
1 (15-ounce) can low-sodium pinto
   beans, rinsed and drained
¼ cup low-sodium chicken broth
½ teaspoon cumin
½ teaspoon coriander
¼ teaspoon chili powder
¼ teaspoon salt
¼ teaspoon pepper
1 tablespoon vegetable oil
½ red onion, sliced into wedges
1 red pepper, cut into strips
1 yellow squash, sliced
8 corn tortillas, warmed
   Cilantro leaves and lime wedges
   for garnish

1. Combine lime juice and zest, cilantro, garlic, and jalapeño in a large resealable plastic bag. Add steak and shake to coat; marinate in refrigerator for 1 hour and up to 8. Remove from refrigerator, scrape off excess marinade, and set aside.

2. Place beans, broth, and spices (through pepper) in a small saucepan and bring to a boil. Reduce heat and simmer 2 minutes. Remove from heat and mash until chunky. Cover and keep warm.

3. Heat a cast-iron skillet over high heat. Add steak and cook until a crust forms and meat is medium-rare, 6–7 minutes per side. Remove from heat and let rest. Slice into ¼-inch-thick slices and keep warm. Heat oil in skillet over high heat, add onion and cook, stirring, until charred, 4–5 minutes. Add peppers and squash and cook, stirring occasionally, until charred, 5–6 minutes.

4. Divide vegetables and steak among 4 plates and serve with ⅓ cup refried beans and 2 tortillas. Garnish with cilantro leaves and lime wedges.

Serving size: 2 tortillas, 4 ounces steak, 1 cup veggies, and ⅓ cup refried beans Calories 414; Fat 11.3g (sat 2.8g, mono 3.3g, poly 3.1g); Cholesterol 70mg; Protein 33g; Carbohydrate 45g; Sugars 3g; Fiber 9g; RS 2.9g; Sodium 236mg

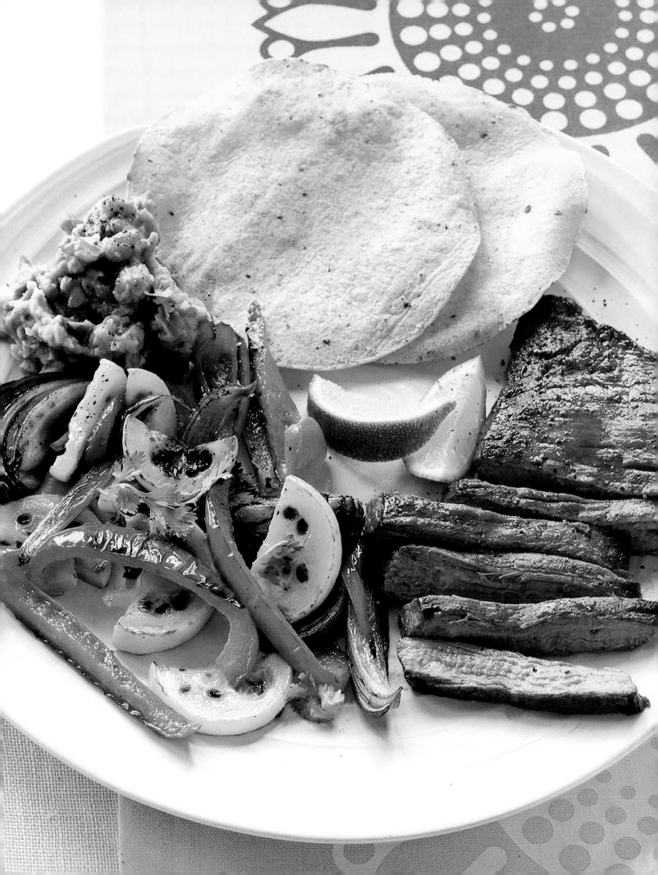

Steak Frites

Prep: 10 minutes | *Cook:* 35 minutes | *Total time:* 45 minutes | *Makes:* 4 servings

We love the simplicity of brasserie-style fare, and it doesn't get much better than steak and fries. We kept the skin on our frites for extra fiber and nutrients.

RS 2.6g

2 pounds Russet potatoes, skin-on
2 tablespoons olive oil
¾ teaspoon salt, divided
1 (1½-pound) hanger steak, trimmed of additional fat
1 teaspoon cracked black pepper
4 teaspoons chopped parsley

1. Preheat oven to 475°. Cut potatoes into ⅓-inch-thick fries. Toss in a bowl with oil and ¼ teaspoon salt. Arrange in a single layer on a large rimmed baking sheet and bake for 20 minutes. Remove from oven. Using a metal spatula, turn fries, lifting carefully so as not to separate crisped parts from potatoes. Return to oven and roast until crisp and golden brown, an additional 15 minutes.

2. While fries are baking, preheat a grill or grill pan over medium-high heat. Season steak with ¼ teaspoon salt and the cracked pepper; grill until medium-rare, 7–8 minutes per side. Remove from heat, let rest, and slice into 4 equal portions

3. Arrange each steak on a dinner plate. Remove fries from oven and season with remaining ¼ teaspoon salt. Place ¼ of fries on each plate and sprinkle with 1 teaspoon chopped parsley.

Serving size: 4 ounces steak and about 15 fries Calories 463; Fat 18.4g (sat 5.4g, mono 10.9g, poly 1.2g); Cholesterol 96mg; Protein 34g; Carbohydrate 40g; Sugars 2g; Fiber 4g; RS 2.6g; Sodium 531mg

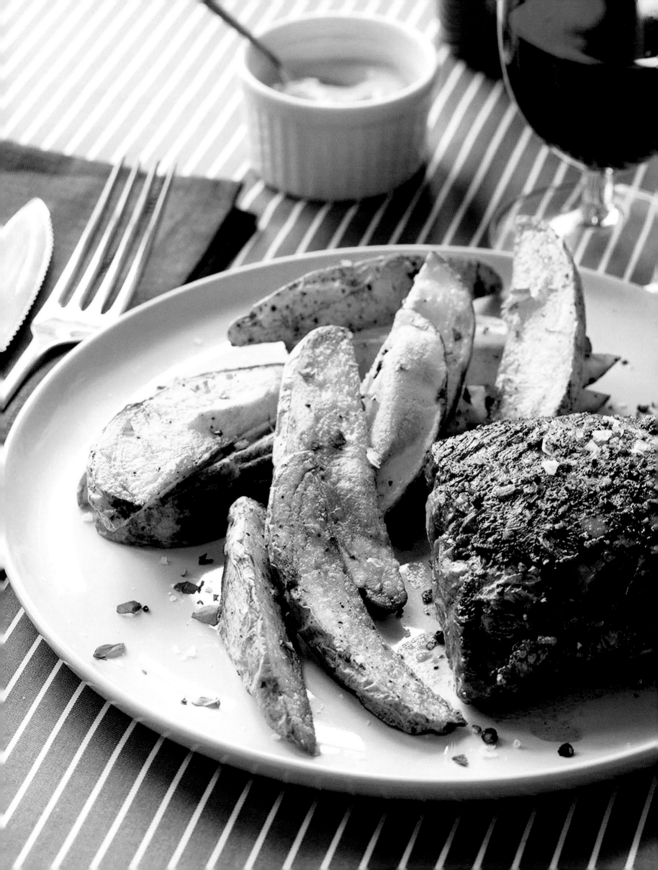

Asian Burger

Southwestern Burger

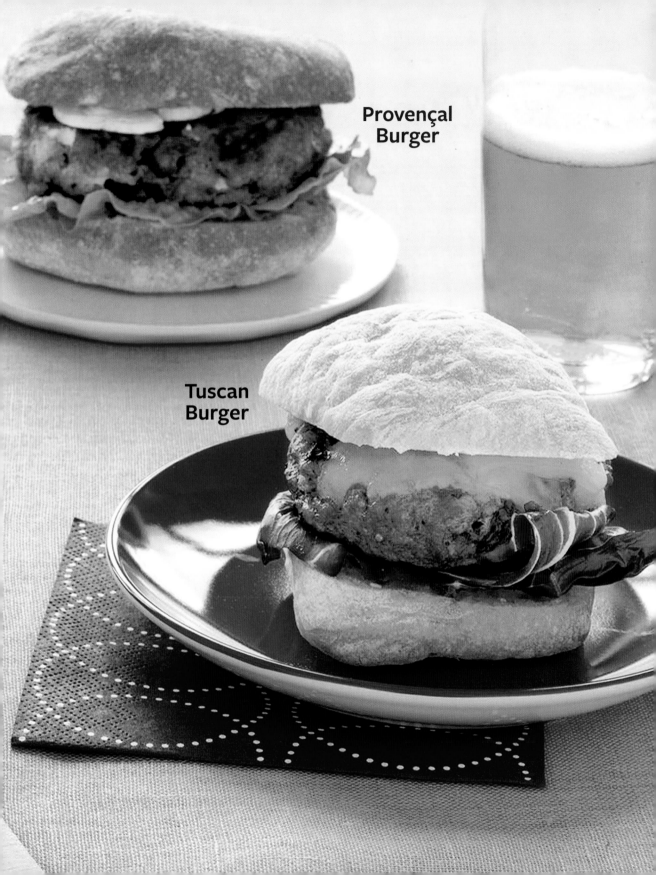

Provençal
Burger

Tuscan
Burger

RS
0.2–2.5g

Dressed-Up Burgers

Prep: *15 minutes* | **Cook:** *10–12 minutes* | **Total time:** *25 minutes* | **Makes:** *4 servings*

There's nothing like sinking your teeth into a juicy burger. To keep it interesting during grilling season, we came up with variations to please every palate, from mild to wild.

BURGER BASE:

- 1 pound extra-lean ground beef
- 1 egg
- ¼ cup finely chopped red onion
- 2 teaspoons finely minced garlic

Serving size: 1 burger, 1 bun, and ¼ toppings

SOUTHWESTERN MIX-INS

- ½ cup frozen corn kernels
- 2 tablespoons chopped cilantro
- ¼ teaspoon chipotle chile powder

Cheese: 4 (¾-ounce) slices Pepper Jack
Lettuce: 4 red-leaf lettuce leaves
Garnish: 8 red onion rings
Bun: 4 plain burger buns

Serving size: 1 burger, 1 bun, and ¼ toppings Calories 399; Fat 15.4g (sat 7.1g, mono 3.2g, poly 1.4g); Cholesterol 131mg; Protein 34g; Carbohydrate 31g; Sugars 5g; Fiber 2g; RS 0.2g; Sodium 414mg

ASIAN MIX-INS

- ¼ cup chopped scallion
- 1 tablespoon toasted sesame seeds

- 2 teaspoons toasted sesame oil
- 1 teaspoon Sriracha

SRIRACHA MAYO FOR BUNS

- 4 tablespoons light mayo
- 2 teaspoons Sriracha sauce

Lettuce: 4 butter lettuce leaves
Bun: 4 sesame seed buns

Serving size: 1 burger, 1 bun, and ¼ toppings Calories 428; Fat 18g (sat 5.1g, mono 5.2g, poly 4.6g); Cholesterol 114mg; Protein 30g; Carbohydrate 36g; Sugars 6g; Fiber 2g; RS 0.5g; Sodium 560mg

TUSCAN MIX-INS

- ½ cup drained, rinsed cannellini beans
- 2 tablespoons minced sundried tomatoes
- 2 tablespoons finely chopped fresh rosemary
- ½ cup chopped arugula

Lettuce for bun: 4 radicchio leaves
Cheese: 4 (¾-ounce) slices Fontina
Bun: 4 square rolls

Serving size: 1 burger, 1 bun, and ¼ toppings Calories 467; Fat 14.4g (sat 7g, mono 4.6g, poly 1g); Cholesterol 133mg; Protein 37g; Carbohydrates 45g; Sugars 3g; Fiber 4g; RS 2.5g; Sodium 685mg

PROVENÇAL MIX-INS

- 1 tablespoon chopped Niçoise olives
- 2 teaspoons dried herbes de Provence

Cheese: ¼ cup goat cheese
Lettuce: 4 Romaine lettuce leaves
Bun: 4 sourdough rolls

Serving size: 1 burger, 1 bun, and ¼ toppings Calories 447; Fat 11g (sat 4.4g, mono 4g, poly 1.4g); Cholesterol 112mg; Protein 35g; Carbohydrate 51g; Sugars 3g; Fiber 3g; RS 1.8g; Sodium 625mg

1. With clean hands, combine base plus mix-in ingredients in a large bowl, then form into 4 equal-size patties. Heat a grill or grill pan over medium-high heat and grill burgers until medium-rare, 5–6 minutes per side. Transfer to a large plate.

2. If recipe calls for cheese, immediately place on top of cooked burger. Place on bun and add additional toppings.

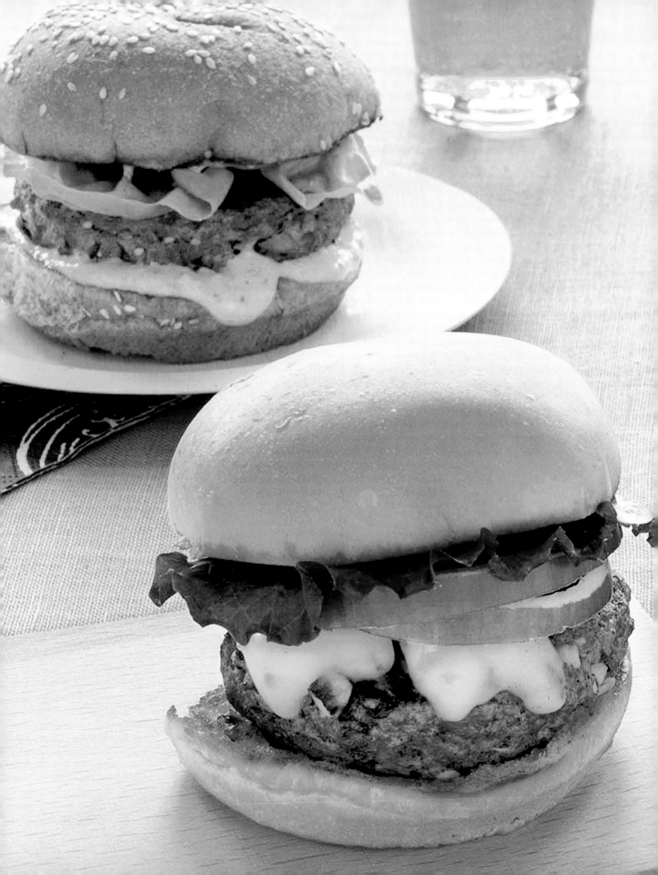

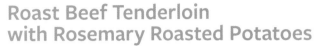

RS
1g

Roast Beef Tenderloin with Rosemary Roasted Potatoes

Prep: 15 minutes | **Cook:** 1 hour | **Total time:** 1 hour 15 minutes | **Makes:** 8 servings

Classic and satisfying, a Sunday roast fills your house with the most amazing aroma. We promise that this will become a family favorite.

2 pounds baby red potatoes, halved
1 tablespoon plus 1 teaspoon olive oil
1 tablespoon chopped fresh rosemary
1¾ teaspoons kosher salt, divided
½ plus ⅛ teaspoon freshly ground black pepper, divided
2 garlic cloves
1 (2½-pound) center-cut beef tenderloin, trimmed
1 (14.5-ounce) can reduced-sodium beef broth
1 tablespoon cornstarch
½ cup dry red wine
1 tablespoon cold butter

1. Preheat oven to 400°. Toss potatoes with 1 tablespoon oil and rosemary on a rimmed baking sheet; season with 1 teaspoon salt and ¼ teaspoon pepper. Roast 10 minutes. (Potatoes will roast 45–60 minutes total.)

2. Meanwhile, finely chop garlic; sprinkle with ½ teaspoon salt. Using flat edge of knife, smash salt and garlic to form a paste. Transfer to a bowl; combine with 1 teaspoon oil and ¼ teaspoon pepper. Rub beef with mixture.

3. Heat a large skillet over high heat. Add beef to skillet, turning occasionally, until browned all over, 5–8 minutes. Remove baking sheet from oven; nestle beef among potatoes. (Reserve skillet.) Roast beef with potatoes until internal temperature reaches 125°, about 30–35 minutes. Transfer roast to a cutting board to rest; continue roasting potatoes until tender, about 10 minutes.

4. Return reserved skillet to heat; add broth, stirring to loosen browned bits. Simmer until reduced by half, 5–8 minutes. Whisk together cornstarch and red wine; add to skillet. Simmer until thickened, 2 minutes. Remove from heat and swirl in butter; season with remaining ¼ teaspoon salt and ⅛ teaspoon pepper. Slice roast and serve with potatoes and sauce.

Serving size: 4 ounces beef, 2½ ounces potatoes, 2 tablespoons sauce Calories 335; Fat 11.7g (sat 4.3g, mono 5.2g, poly 0.6g); Cholesterol 81mg; Protein 30g; Carbohydrate 23g; Sugars 2g; Fiber 2g; RS 1g; Sodium 581mg

Slow-Baked BBQ Ribs

Prep: *10 minutes* | **Cook:** *3 hours 10 minutes* | **Total time:** *3 hours 20 minutes*
Makes: *6 appetizer-size servings*

Succulent, juicy, and super-saucy, our BBQ ribs are much lower in fat than a traditional version. Definitely don't wear white when you eat them!

¼ cup no-salt-added tomato sauce
1 tablespoon mustard
1 tablespoon brown sugar
1 tablespoon chili powder
1 teaspoon apple cider vinegar
½ teaspoon cumin
¼ teaspoon salt
½ teaspoon smoked paprika
¼ teaspoon cayenne pepper
1½ pounds 3-inch beef spare ribs
(about 6 pieces), trimmed of
visible fat

1. Combine first 9 ingredients (through cayenne) in a small bowl; reserve barbecue sauce.

2. Preheat broiler. Place ribs on a rimmed baking sheet and broil until browned, 5 minutes per side. Remove ribs from oven and tip fat from baking sheet; discard. Cool ribs for 15 minutes. Meanwhile, preheat oven to 300°.

3. Place ribs in a square baking dish and spread barbecue sauce on ribs. Wrap tightly in foil and bake until fork-tender, about 3 hours. Drain additional fat from baking dish and serve ribs while hot.

Serving size: 1 spare rib Calories 306; Fat 23.1g (sat 9.3g, mono 9.8g, poly 1g); Cholesterol 70mg; Protein 19g; Carbohydrate 4g; Sugars 3g; Fiber 1g; RS 0g; Sodium 205mg

RS
1.3g

Chili Dogs

Prep: *15 minutes* | **Cook:** *19 minutes* | **Total time:** *34 minutes* | **Makes:** *4 servings*

☺

Break out the extra napkins! Our loaded chili dogs are absolutely packed with toppings—and totally delicious. You'll have chili left over, which is great on its own or served over a baked potato.

CHILI:

- 2 teaspoons olive oil
- 1 small onion, diced (1 cup)
- 2 minced garlic cloves
- 1 (15-ounce) can low-sodium kidney beans, rinsed and drained
- 1 (8-ounce) can low-sodium tomato sauce
- 1 teaspoon chili powder
- ¼ teaspoon salt
- ¼ teaspoon pepper
- 4 low-fat hot dogs, grilled
- 4 hot dog buns

TOPPINGS:

- ¼ cup diced tomato
- ¼ cup diced red onion
- ¼ cup reduced-fat cheddar cheese
- ¼ cup diced green chiles

1. Make chili: Heat oil in a small saucepan over medium-high heat. Add onion and cook, stirring, until soft and translucent, 6–7 minutes, Add garlic and cook 1 minute. Add beans, tomato sauce, ¼ cup water, chili powder, salt, and pepper. Bring to a boil, then reduce heat and cook, stirring occasionally, until beans absorb some of the liquid and chili has thickened, 12–15 minutes.

2. Place a hot dog on a hot dog bun. Top with ¼ cup chili, and 1 tablespoon each of tomato, onion, cheese, and chiles.

Serving size: 1 hot dog, ¼ cup chili, 1 tablespoon each tomato, onion, cheese, and chiles   Calories 340; Fat 13g (sat 4.3g, mono 0.8g, poly 0.2g); Cholesterol 35mg; Protein 17g; Carbohydrate 38g; Sugars 9g; Fiber 7g; RS 1.3g; Sodium 811mg

TIP:
To lower the risk of choking, please be sure to cut hot dogs into small pieces for young children.

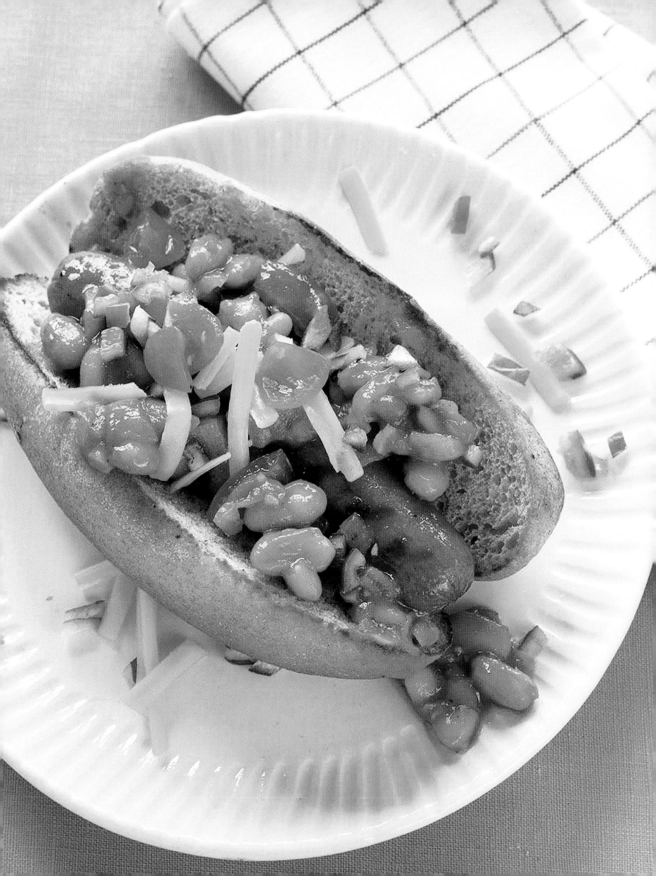

RS
0.6g

Grilled Chicken Cutlets with Summer Succotash

Prep time: *1 minute* | **Cook time:** *4 minutes* | **Total time:** *5 minutes* | **Makes:** *4 servings*

A main dish in 5 minutes flat? It's doable when you use frozen vegetables and ultrathin chicken cutlets.

4	chicken cutlets (1 pound total)
¼	teaspoon kosher salt
¼	teaspoon freshly ground black pepper
1	tablespoon olive oil
½	cup frozen corn, thawed
1	cup frozen baby lima beans, thawed
1	pint grape tomatoes
1	tablespoon grated Parmesan
½	cup fresh basil leaves, torn if large
	Lemon wedges for serving

1. Heat a grill pan over high heat; season chicken cutlets with salt and pepper. Cook chicken cutlets until cooked through, 3–4 minutes, turning once.

2. Meanwhile, heat oil in a large skillet over medium-high heat. Add corn, lima beans, and grape tomatoes to skillet. Cook, tossing occasionally, until tomatoes begin to burst, 3–4 minutes. Stir Parmesan and basil into pan and divide mixture among plates. Top with cooked chicken; serve with lemon wedges.

Serving size: 1 chicken cutlet and ¾ cup vegetables
Calories 265; Fat 7.1g (sat1.6g, mono 3.7g, poly 1.2g); Cholesterol 73mg; Protein 31g; Carbohydrate 18g; Sugars 4g; Fiber 4g; RS 0.6g; Sodium 216mg

> **TIP:**
> Pump up the Resistant Starch in this meal by adding a whole wheat or rye roll.

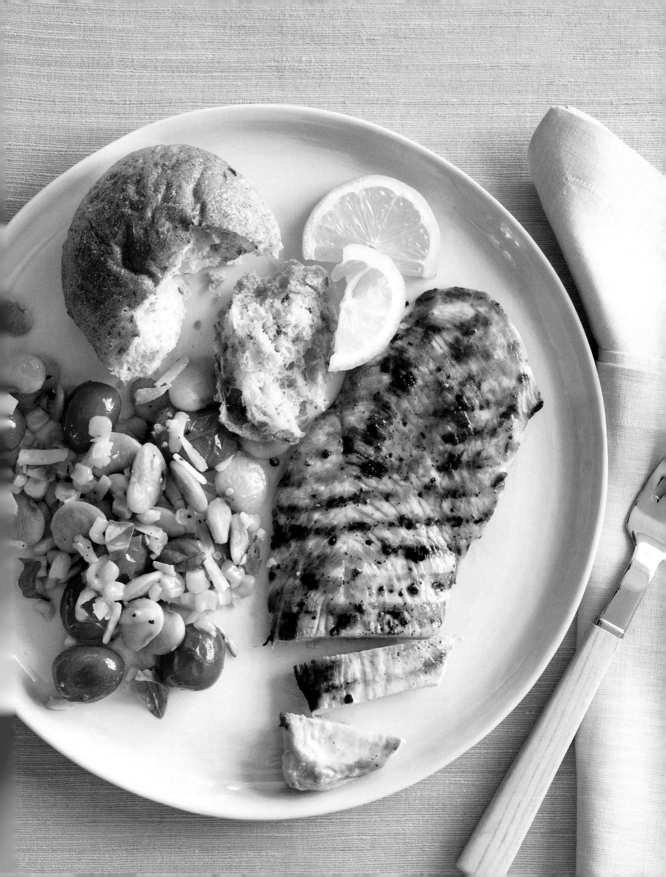

RS
0.9g

Cornflake-Crusted Chicken Tenders

Prep: *25 minutes* | **Cook:** *12 minutes* | **Total time:** *37 minutes* | **Makes:** *4 servings*

Kids of all ages love fried chicken fingers. We lightened up this recipe by using Resistant Starch–filled cornflakes to coat the chicken, and then baked them to cut the fat. Go on—they're not just for kids anymore!

- 4 cups cornflakes
- 1 tablespoon sesame seeds
- ½ teaspoon paprika, divided
- ¼ teaspoon salt
- ½ teaspoon pepper, divided
- ¼ teaspoon cayenne pepper
- ¼ cup all purpose flour
- 4 (4-ounce) boneless, skinless chicken breasts, pounded to ½-inch thickness
- 2 egg whites, lightly beaten
  Olive oil cooking spray

1. Preheat oven to 400°.

2. Place cornflakes in a food processor and pulse to make 1 cup crumbs, 20–30 seconds. Combine cornflake crumbs, sesame seeds, ¼ teaspoon each paprika, salt and pepper, and cayenne in a shallow dish.

3. Place flour and remaining paprika and pepper in a resealable plastic bag and shake gently to mix.

4. Place egg whites in another shallow dish.

5. Slice each chicken breast into 6 strips and place in bag with flour and shake well to coat.

6. In batches, place coated chicken strips in egg whites. Remove, shaking off excess, and roll in cornflake-crumb mixture.

7. Arrange coated tenders on a baking sheet and coat tops of tenders lightly with cooking spray.

8. Bake until crisp and golden, 11–12 minutes.

Serving size: 6 tenders Calories 284; Fat 4.7g (sat 0.9g, mono 1.5g, poly 1.2g); Cholesterol 73mg; Protein 29g; Carbohydrate 31g; Sugars 3g; Fiber 1g; RS 0.9g; Sodium 508mg

Lemon-Herb Roasted Turkey Breast

Prep: *10 minutes* | **Cook:** *1 hour 30 minutes + resting* | **Total time:** *1 hour 40 minutes* | **Makes:** *6 servings*

There's no reason to spend hours cooking a whole turkey when you can make this juicy turkey breast in half the time. Serve with roasted new potatoes or our Herb and Olive Oil Mashed Potatoes on page 194.

2 tablespoons olive oil
1 tablespoon chopped rosemary
1 tablespoon chopped thyme
1 tablespoon chopped oregano
1 lemon, zested; reserve zest and lemon
1 minced large garlic clove
½ teaspoon salt
½ teaspoon cracked black pepper
1 (2½-pound) bone-in skinless turkey breast, patted dry
⅓ cup dry white wine

1. Preheat oven to 350°.

2. Combine oil, rosemary, thyme, oregano, zest, garlic, salt, and pepper in a small bowl to form a paste. Spread evenly over turkey breast. Place in a roasting pan and gently pour wine into bottom of pan.

3. Slice zested lemon into wedges and place in bottom of pan. Tent with foil and roast for 1 hour. Remove foil and continue roasting until an instant-read thermometer reads 165°, about 30–40 minutes. Remove from oven and let turkey rest for 10 minutes.

4. Transfer to a cutting board and slice off the bone into ½-inch-thick slices. Squeeze roasted lemons into pan juices and pour 2 tablespoons pan juices onto each portion.

Serving size: 4 ounces turkey and 2 tablespoons sauce
Calories 236; Fat 5.6g (sat 1g, mono 3.5g, poly 0.8g); Cholesterol 110mg; Protein 40g; Carbohydrate 3g; Sugars 0g; Fiber 1g; RS 0g; Sodium 264mg

Individual Chicken Pot Pies

Prep time: 20 minutes | **Cook Time:** 1 hour 15 minutes | **Total:** 1 hour 35 minutes | **Makes:** 4 servings

The flaky crust on our chicken pot pie is so inviting, you'll hardly be able to resist digging in. This may be the ultimate comfort recipe.

1 tablespoon olive oil
1 small onion, chopped (1 cup)
2 minced garlic cloves
1 tablespoon chopped fresh thyme
1 cup diced celery
1 cup diced carrots
1 pound boneless, skinless chicken breasts, diced
¼ cup white wine
⅓ cup flour
3 cups milk
1 cup low-sodium chicken broth
2 teaspoons Worcestershire sauce
¼ teaspoon salt
¼ teaspoon pepper
1 cup frozen peas
6 sheets frozen phyllo dough, thawed
   Olive oil cooking spray

1. Preheat oven to 400°.

2. Heat oil in a medium saucepan over medium-high heat and cook onion, stirring occasionally, until soft and translucent, 6–7 minutes. Add garlic and thyme and cook 1 minute. Add celery and carrots and cook until crisp-tender, 2–3 minutes. Add chicken and cook, stirring occasionally, until no longer pink and cooked through, 5–6 minutes.

3. Add wine; cook until mostly absorbed, 2–3 minutes. Add flour to pan; cook, stirring, for 2 minutes. Whisk in milk, broth, Worcestershire sauce, salt, and pepper. Bring to a boil, reduce heat, and cook, whisking, until mixture thickens, 15 minutes. Add peas during last minute. Remove from heat and reserve.

4. Arrange 6 sheets of stacked phyllo dough on a surface. Place a 5-inch bowl on the bottom right quarter of the stacked sheets. Using a pizza cutter, cut around the bowl to form a circle. Coat on top and in between layers lightly with cooking spray. Using the pizza cutter, cut 3 (½-inch) slits into the phyllo round. Repeat with remaining dough. Place four 5-inch ovensafe bowls on a rimmed baking sheet. Pour 1¾ cups mixture into each; transfer phyllo rounds to cover, pressing gently. Bake until tops are browned, 35–40 minutes. Remove from oven and serve hot.

Serving size: 1 pot pie Calories 455; Fat 9.8g (sat 2.8g, mono 4.7g, poly 1.4g); Cholesterol 76mg; Protein 39g; Carbohydrate 49g; Sugars 16g; Fiber 7g; RS 1.6g; Sodium 551mg

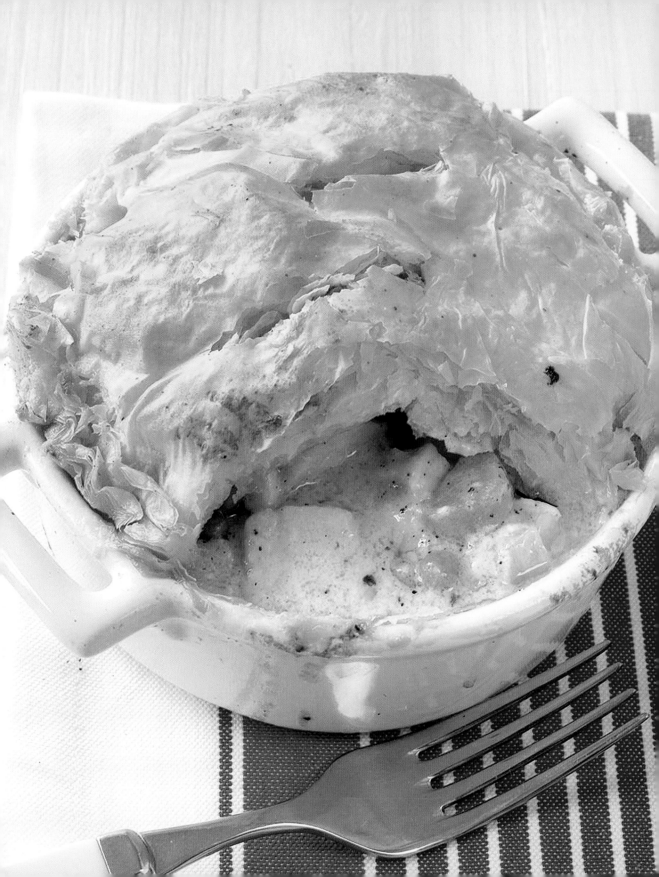

Orange Chicken Stir-Fry

Prep: 10 minutes | **Cook:** 35 minutes | **Total:** 45 minutes | **Makes:** 4 servings

If you're a fan of Chinese takeout, give this healthy, superlow-sodium version a spin. It will probably be on the table faster than your local joint can deliver.

2 navel oranges, cut into segments (1 cup), membranes squeezed to make ¼ cup juice
2 tablespoons rice wine vinegar
1 teaspoon finely grated ginger
1 garlic clove, finely grated
¼ teaspoon crushed red pepper
2 scallions, sliced, whites and greens separated
2 (6-ounce) boneless, skinless chicken breasts, thinly sliced
1 cup brown rice
2 teaspoons vegetable oil
¼ cup sliced almonds
2 bunches watercress (10 ounces), thick stems removed
1 teaspoon sesame oil

1. Whisk together orange juice, vinegar, ginger, garlic, crushed red pepper, and scallion whites in a large shallow bowl. Add chicken and marinate in the refrigerator for at least 20 minutes and up to 1 hour.

2. Meanwhile, cook rice according to package directions.

3. Heat oil in a large heavy skillet over medium-high heat. With a slotted spoon, remove chicken from marinade and transfer to hot skillet. Cook chicken about 3 minutes or until partially cooked through; stir in almonds and watercress. Cook, stirring, until watercress is wilted and chicken is cooked, 1 minute more. Gently toss orange segments and sesame oil into stir-fry; serve over rice.

Serving size: About 4 ounces stir-fry, ½ cup cooked rice
Calories 378; Fat 10.1g (sat 1.3g, mono 3.9g, poly 3.6g); Cholesterol 54mg; Protein 26g; Carbohydrate 47g; Sugars 7g; Fiber 6g; RS 2.7g; Sodium 135mg

Herbed Turkey-Feta Burgers

Prep: 15 minutes | **Cook:** 15 minutes (*including assembly*) | **Total time:** 30 minutes | **Makes:** 4 servings

Greek spices, feta cheese, and zesty yogurt dip make this the tastiest turkey burger you've ever tried. Use ground turkey breast to lower the fat even more.

1	pound ground turkey
½	teaspoon freshly ground black pepper
¼	cup crumbled feta cheese
¼	cup diced roasted red pepper
¼	cup diced red onion
2	tablespoons finely chopped parsley
2	teaspoons finely chopped oregano
4	(½-inch) onion ring slices
½	cup lowfat Greek yogurt
2	tablespoons lemon juice
1	teaspoon lemon zest
⅛	teaspoon salt
⅛	teaspoon pepper
4	whole grain burger buns, split
4	lettuce leaves

1. Combine turkey, pepper, feta, roasted red pepper, red onion, parsley, and oregano in a large bowl; form into 4 equal-size patties. Chill until ready to use.

2. Coat a grill or grill pan with cooking spray and heat over medium-high heat. Grill burgers until cooked through, 5 minutes per side. When cooking second side of burgers, grill onions until charred, about 5 minutes. Whisk together yogurt, lemon juice, zest, salt, and pepper. Spread 2 tablespoons yogurt dressing on the bottom of a bun. Place one lettuce leaf and one grilled onion ring on it. Top with a burger and other half of bun.

Serving size: 1 bun, 1 burger, 1 lettuce leaf, and 1 grilled onion ring Calories 370; Fat 13.7g (sat 4.4g, mono 4.1g, poly 3.4g); Cholesterol 85mg; Protein 31g; Carbohydrate 34g; Sugars 9g; Fiber 5g; RS 0.4g; Sodium 441mg

Sides & Salads

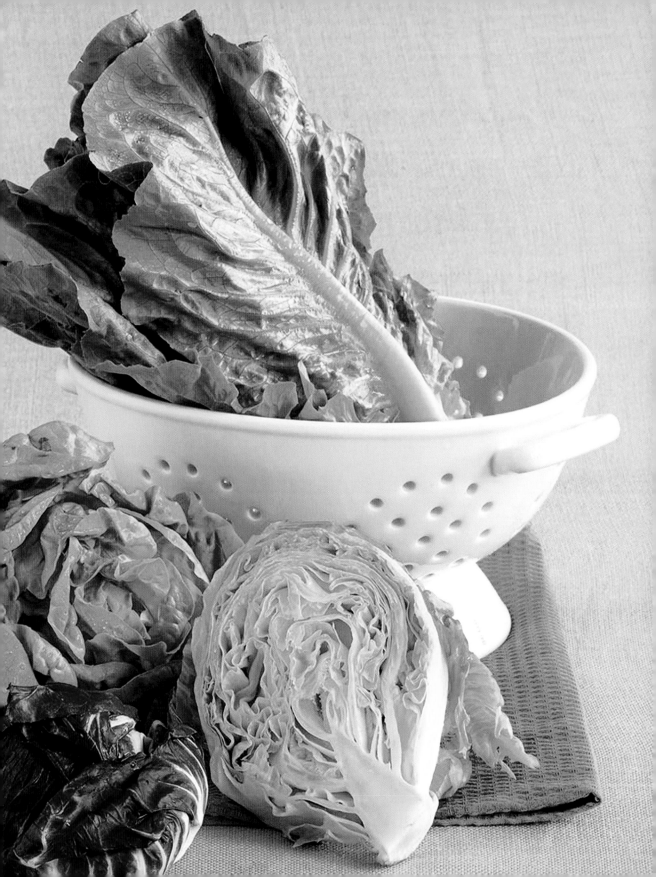

RS
3g

Barley Salad with Corn, Feta, Basil, and Charred Tomatoes

Prep: *5 minutes* | ***Cook:*** *20 minutes* | ***Total time:*** *25 minutes* | ***Makes:*** *4 servings*

Flavorful, colorful, and full of Resistant Starch, this healthy salad is a wonderful side dish for chicken or steak, and makes a fantastic vegetarian entrée.

1   cup pearl barley
1   cup frozen corn
1   pint grape tomatoes
3   tablespoons olive oil, divided
1   tablespoon white-wine vinegar
½   teaspoon salt, divided
¼   teaspoon freshly ground black pepper
½   cup crumbled feta cheese
¼   cup sliced basil leaves

1. Preheat broiler with rack in highest position. Cover barley with salted water in a medium saucepan and cook over medium heat until just tender, about 15 minutes. Add corn; remove from heat. Let stand 1 minute; drain and run under cold water until cooled.

2. Meanwhile, toss tomatoes with 1 tablespoon oil; season with ¼ teaspoon salt and pepper. Broil, tossing occasionally, until tomatoes become charred and they burst, about 8 minutes.

3. Whisk together vinegar and remaining 2 tablespoons oil in a medium bowl; season with remaining ¼ teaspoon salt. Add barley and corn to bowl and toss with dressing; fold in tomatoes, feta, and basil.

Serving size: 1¼ cups salad Calories 340; Fat 14.9g (sat 4.4g, mono 8.4g, poly 1.6g); Cholesterol 17mg; Protein 7g; Carbohydrate 46g; Sugars 5g; Fiber 6g; RS 3g; Sodium 562mg

> **TIP**
> Barley is loaded with Resistant Starch and makes a delicious, filling side dish. Cook extra and refrigerate for up to 4 days or freeze for up to 3 months in a freezer-safe bag or container. Squeeze out all the air before freezing, and mark with the cook date.

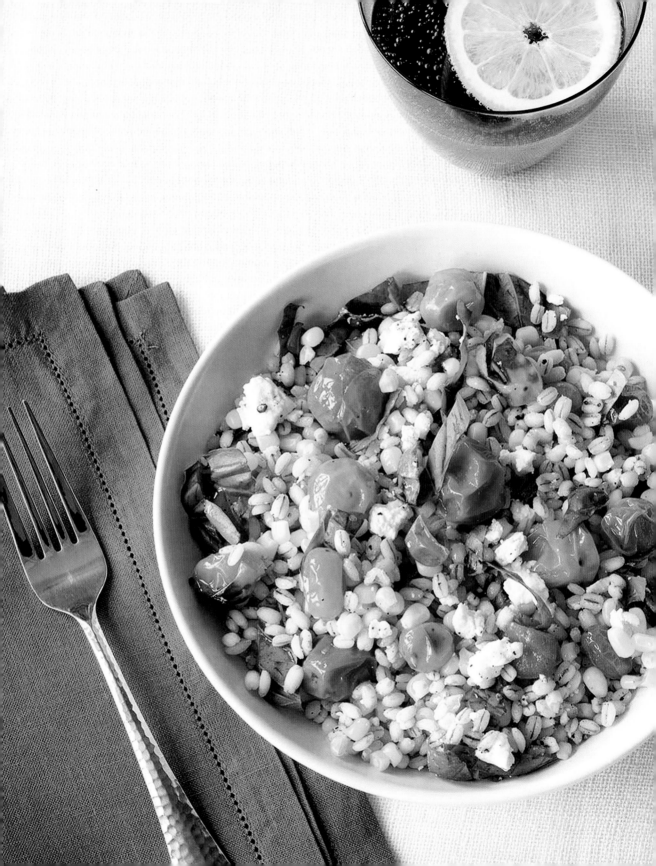

Thai Green Mango Salad with Rotisserie Chicken

Prep: *10 minutes* | **Total time:** *10 minutes* | **Makes:** *4 servings*

Refreshing and light, this salad is perfect for warm summer nights. And it's a great way to use leftover chicken.

1 tablespoon chile-garlic sauce (such as Sriracha)
¼ cup fresh lime juice
1 tablespoon fish sauce
2 tablespoons brown sugar
1 unripe mango (about 1 pound), peeled and thinly sliced
1 cup matchstick carrots
2 cups shredded chicken (from 3-pound rotisserie chicken)
1 cup cilantro leaves
1 cup halved grape tomatoes
2 tablespoons peanuts, chopped

Whisk together chile-garlic sauce, lime juice, fish sauce, and sugar in a large bowl. Add mango, carrots, chicken, cilantro, and tomatoes; toss. Sprinkle with peanuts before serving.

Serving size: 1¼ cups Calories 265; Fat 7.7g (sat 1.8g, mono 3.1g, poly 1.9g); Cholesterol 63mg; Protein 23g; Carbohydrate 28g; Sugars 22g; Fiber 3g; RS 0g; Sodium 352mg

ASK CARBLOVERS

Q: **Can I eat all the veggies and salads I want on *CarbLovers*?**

A: We love veggies and salads on this diet! Feel free to add a green side salad with a tablespoon of vinaigrette to any meal. Vegetables are high in fiber and water and help you feel full between meals, but you can overdo the calories once you start adding toppings and dressing.

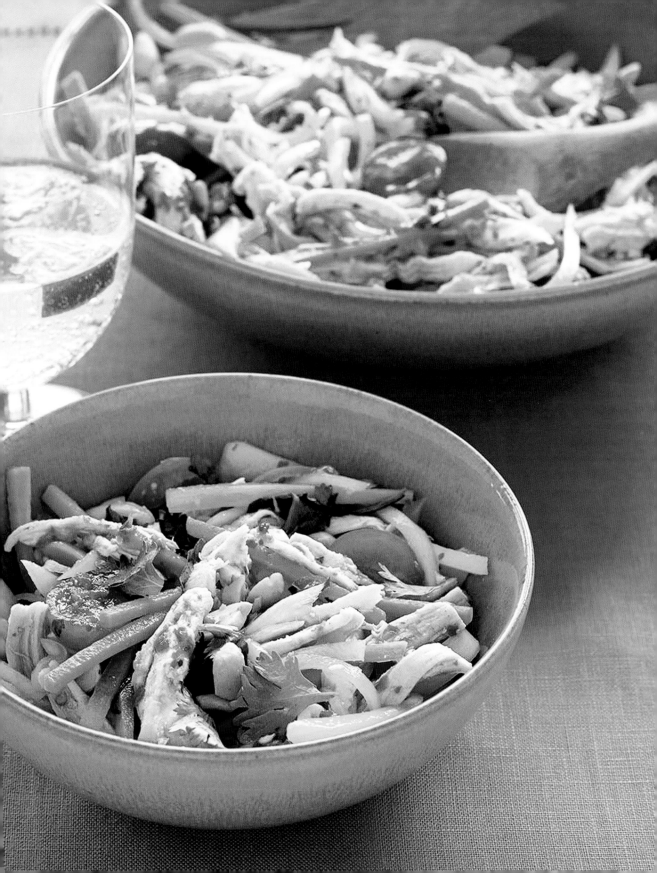

Creamy Cobb Salad

Grilled Chicken Caesar Salad with Pumpernickel Croutons

Niçoise Salad

Salmon
Waldorf
Salad

Creamy Cobb Salad

Prep: *15 minutes* | **Cook:** *5 minutes* | **Total time:** *20 minutes* | **Makes:** *4 servings*

Salads can sometimes taste a bit boring. Not this one. We've taken a traditional Cobb and lightened it up, but it's still packed with flavor.

FOR DRESSING:

⅓ cup low-fat buttermilk
3 tablespoons light sour cream
2 tablespoons light mayonnaise
1 tablespoon red wine vinegar
1 teaspoon Dijon mustard
1 teaspoon freshly ground black pepper

FOR SALAD:

4 slices (3 ounces) Canadian bacon, diced
5 cups chopped iceberg lettuce
3 cups chopped radicchio
8 ounces thick-cut roasted turkey breast, diced
2 cups cherry tomatoes, halved
½ avocado, diced (about ½ cup)
¼ cup chopped red onion
2 hard-boiled eggs, chopped

MAKE DRESSING:

Whisk together dressing ingredients in a small bowl. Cover and refrigerate until ready to use.

MAKE SALAD:

1. Coat a large nonstick pan with cooking spray and heat over medium-high heat. Add bacon and cook until crisp, 4–5 minutes. Remove from pan and reserve.

2. Toss together lettuce and radicchio in a large bowl; divide among 4 salad bowls. Top each with ¼ of the bacon, turkey, tomatoes, avocado, onion, and eggs. Drizzle each salad with about 2½ tablespoons dressing; toss and serve.

Serving size: 1 salad Calories 279; Fat 12.1g (sat 3.1g, mono 4.4g, poly 2.6g); Cholesterol 158mg; Protein 29g; Carbohydrate 15g; Sugars 7g; Fiber 4g; RS 0g; Sodium 499mg

TIP
If you follow a gluten-free diet, check the ingredient list on your mayo; some contain gluten. Go to celiac.org for more info.

Grilled Chicken Caesar Salad with Pumpernickel Croutons

Prep: 20 minutes | **Cook:** 10 minutes | **Total time:** 30 minutes | **Makes:** 4 servings

☺

We took a basic Caesar salad and put our CarbLovers *spin on it by adding homemade pumpernickel croutons for more Resistant Starch.*

FOR CROUTONS:

2 thick slices pumpernickel bread, cubed (about 2½ cups)
1 tablespoon olive oil
1 small clove minced garlic
¼ teaspoon pepper

FOR CHICKEN BREASTS:

4 thin-cut skinless boneless chicken breasts (1 pound)
¼ teaspoon salt
¼ teaspoon pepper
¼ teaspoon paprika

FOR DRESSING:

1 raw egg or 3 tablespoons pasteurized egg product
3 tablespoons lemon juice
1 tablespoon water
1 tablespoon finely minced garlic
2 teaspoons Dijon mustard
½ teaspoon cracked black pepper
2 anchovy fillets, drained and mashed (about 2 teaspoons)
¼ cup olive oil

FOR SALAD:

12 cups chopped romaine lettuce
2 vine-ripened tomatoes, cut into wedges
¼ cup coarsely shredded Parmesan cheese (1 ounce)

MAKE CROUTONS:

Preheat oven to 350°. Toss bread, oil, garlic, and pepper in a bowl to coat. Transfer to a rimmed baking sheet; bake until lightly toasted, 8–9 minutes. Remove from oven and cool completely.

MAKE CHICKEN BREASTS:

Preheat a grill or grill pan over medium-high heat. Season chicken with salt, pepper, and paprika; grill until cooked through, 3 minutes per side. Remove from heat, rest, and slice into ½-inch slices on the diagonal.

MAKE DRESSING:

Combine first 7 dressing ingredients in a bowl and whisk to incorporate. Slowly whisk in oil until emulsified and creamy.

MAKE SALAD:

Arrange 3 cups lettuce in each of 4 salad bowls. Add 1 sliced chicken breast, 4 tomato wedges, and ½ cup croutons on top of each salad. Drizzle with 3 tablespoons dressing and garnish with 1 tablespoon Parmesan and additional cracked pepper, if desired.

Serving size: 1 salad Calories 423; Fat 23.7g (sat 4.6g, mono 14.5g, poly 3.3g); Cholesterol 115mg; Protein 32g; Carbohydrate 22g; Sugars 4g; Fiber 6g; RS 1.1g; Sodium 609mg

Salmon Waldorf Salad

Prep: *15 minutes* | **Cook:** *17 minutes* | **Total time:** *32 minutes* | **Makes:** *4 servings*

Creamy dressing and crunchy walnuts are the cornerstones of this main or side-dish salad. We added heart-healthy salmon to boost the good fats in this classic dish.

FOR DRESSING:

- 2 tablespoons light mayonnaise
- 2 tablespoons plain low-fat yogurt
- 2 tablespoons fresh lemon juice
- ½ teaspoon salt, divided
- ½ teaspoon pepper, divided

FOR SALAD:

- 1 pound skinless salmon fillet
- 1 small red apple, diced
- ½ cup seedless red grapes, halved
- 2 stalks celery, finely minced (⅔ cup)
- 2 tablespoons walnuts, coarsely chopped, divided
- 1 head butter lettuce, leaves separated

Preheat oven to 350°.

MAKE DRESSING:

Whisk mayonnaise, yogurt, lemon juice, and ¼ teaspoon each of salt and pepper together in a large bowl. Set aside.

MAKE SALAD:

1. Season salmon with remaining salt and pepper, place on a foil-lined baking sheet; bake until cooked through, 16–17 minutes. Remove from oven, cool, and flake.

2. Add flaked salmon, apples, grapes, celery, and half of the walnuts to the bowl with the dressing. Arrange 4 lettuce leaves in a shallow bowl and top with 1 cup salad. Garnish with remaining walnuts.

Serving size: 1 salad Calories 268; Fat 13.3g (sat 2g, mono 3.7g, poly 6.4g); Cholesterol 75mg; Protein 27g; Carbohydrate 10g; Sugars 7g; Fiber 1g; RS 0g; Sodium 420m

RS
3.2g

Niçoise Salad

Prep: 30 minutes | **Total time:** 30 minutes | **Makes:** 4 servings

This classic French recipe was popularized by none other than Julia Child. Our version is vegetarian, but you could add a 6-ounce can of unsalted tuna back in if you'd like.

FOR DRESSING:

- 1 teaspoon minced shallot
- 1 teaspoon Dijon mustard
- ¼ teaspoon salt
- ¼ teaspoon pepper
- 2 tablespoons fresh lemon juice
- ¼ cup extra virgin olive oil

FOR SALAD:

- 10 cups chopped romaine lettuce leaves
- 4 (4-ounce) red potatoes, steamed and sliced
- 1 cup canned white beans, rinsed and drained
- 4 hard-boiled eggs, halved
- 2 cups lightly steamed green beans
- 2 large vine-ripened tomatoes, cut into wedges
- 16 niçoise olives
- 4 large caperberries, rinsed and drained

MAKE DRESSING:

Whisk together first 5 dressing ingredients in a small bowl. Add oil in a slow stream and whisk to emulsify. Set aside.

MAKE SALAD:

Divide lettuce among 4 salad bowls. Evenly distribute potatoes, beans, eggs, green beans, tomatoes, olives, and caperberries among bowls. Drizzle each salad with about 2½ tablespoons dressing.

Serving size: 1 salad Calories 433; Fat 23.1g (sat 4.1g, mono 14.8g, poly 3.2g); Cholesterol 186mg; Protein 16g; Carbohydrate 44g; Sugars 7g; Fiber 9g; RS 3.2g; Sodium 641mg

Sweet Potato and Black Bean Salad

Prep: 5 minutes | *Cook:* 25 minutes | *Total time:* 30 minutes | *Makes:* 4 servings

Sweet potatoes and black beans score sky-high in antioxidants. Combine them in this simple, filling salad, and you have a power pair!

2   medium sweet potatoes
    (1 pound), cut into ½-inch cubes
1   tablespoon olive oil
½   teaspoon paprika
¼   teaspoon kosher salt
¼   teaspoon pepper
1   (15-ounce) can black beans,
    rinsed and drained
¼   cup chopped fresh cilantro
1   tablespoon lime juice

1. Preheat oven to 400°. Toss potatoes with oil, paprika, salt, and pepper on a large rimmed baking sheet. Roast 20 to 25 minutes, tossing once, or until potatoes are browned in spots and tender.

2. Transfer potatoes to a large bowl with beans, cilantro, and lime juice; toss to combine. Serve warm.

Serving size: 1 cup Calories 184; Fat 3.9g (sat 0.6g, mono 2.5g, poly 0.6g); Cholesterol 0mg; Protein 7g; Carbohydrate 32g; Sugars 5g; Fiber 8g; RS 2g; Sodium 297mg

TIP:
Add 12 ounces grilled shrimp or chicken to turn this into a delicious protein-packed meal for four.

RS
1.1g

Warm Potato and Spinach Salad

Prep: 5 minutes | **Cook:** 20 minutes | **Total time:** 25 minutes | **Makes:** 6 servings

This delicious side will become your new picnic go-to. The salty prosciutto and tangy vinaigrette are a winning combination.

1¼ pounds red new potatoes
2 tablespoons olive oil
2 tablespoons white balsamic vinegar
¼ teaspoon salt
¼ teaspoon pepper
3 cups baby spinach
2 ounces prosciutto, pulled into pieces

1. Place potatoes in a medium saucepan and cover with water. Bring to a boil. Reduce heat and simmer 20 minutes. Cut potatoes into quarters.

2. Whisk oil and vinegar in a large bowl to combine; season with salt and pepper. Add warm potatoes, spinach, and prosciutto to dressing; toss to combine and serve.

Serving size: about 1 cup Calories 138; Fat 5.6g (sat 1g, mono 3.3g, poly 0.5g); Cholesterol 7mg; Protein 5g; Carbohydrate 19g; Sugars 1g; Fiber 2g; RS 1.1g; Sodium 374mg

10 POINTS

**RS
2.9g**

Broccoli and Cheese–Stuffed Baked Potato

Prep: *10 minutes* | **Cook:** *13 minutes to 70 minutes, depending on method*
Total time: *23 minutes (microwave)* | **Makes:** *4 servings*

When was the last time you indulged in a cheesy baked potato? Well, it's on the menu again, and this one is nutrition-packed!

4	large Idaho potatoes, scrubbed
¾	cup skim milk
1	tablespoon flour
4	ounces reduced-fat extra-sharp cheddar cheese (1 cup), shredded
½	teaspoon salt
¼	teaspoon pepper
⅛	teaspoon cayenne pepper
1	(10-ounce) package frozen broccoli florets, defrosted

1. Cook potatoes:

OVEN: Preheat oven to 400°. Pierce potatoes with a fork, and wrap each in foil. Bake until tender, 1 hour.

MICROWAVE: Pierce potatoes with a fork, and wrap each in a paper towel. Place in microwave, and cook on HIGH 8 minutes, until just tender (test with with a knife; potatoes will continue to cook when removed from microwave).

2. While potatoes are cooking, make sauce: Combine milk and flour in a small saucepan over high heat; bring to a simmer and cook, whisking, until thickened, 2–3 minutes. Add cheese, salt, pepper, and cayenne; whisk until sauce is smooth. Continue to simmer, whisking, 2 minutes.

3. Place broccoli in a microwave-safe dish; microwave on HIGH 4–5 minutes, until hot.

4. Split cooked potatoes open with a knife. Spoon ½ cup broccoli into each potato, and top with ¼ cup cheddar sauce.

Serving size: 1 potato, ½ cup broccoli, and ¼ cup cheddar sauce Calories 377; Fat 5.8g (sat 3.4g, mono 1.4g, poly 0.4g); Cholesterol 17mg; Protein 18g; Carbohydrate 66g; Sugars 6g; Fiber 7g; RS 2.9g; Sodium 403mg

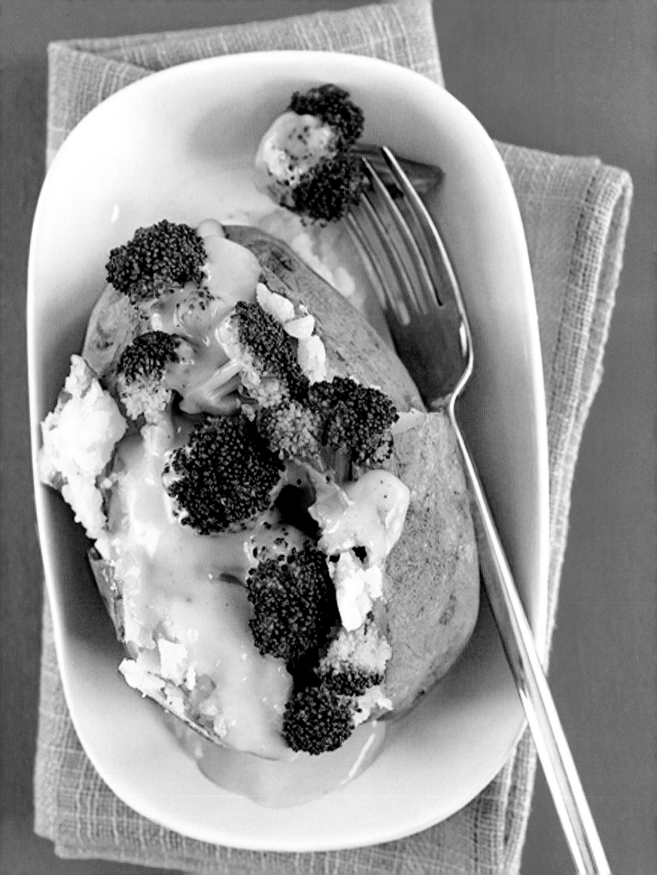

Sweet Potato Fries with Curried Ketchup

Prep: *10 minutes* | **Cook:** *30 minutes* | **Total time:** *40 minutes* | **Makes:** *4 servings*

Everyone loves fries, and our version can be enjoyed guilt-free! Not only are they delicious, but they also provide more than 100% of your daily vitamin A.

2 medium sweet potatoes, scrubbed and dried (about 1 pound), cut into long, ½-inch-thick wedges
1 tablespoon olive oil
½ teaspoon kosher salt, divided
¼ teaspoon freshly ground black pepper
1 tablespoon fresh lime juice
½ cup ketchup
2 teaspoons freshly grated ginger
1½ teaspoons curry powder
⅛ teaspoon cayenne pepper

1. Preheat oven to 400°. Toss potatoes on a large rimmed baking sheet with oil. Season potatoes with ¼ teaspoon of the salt and pepper. Roast 30–40 minutes, tossing once, until charred and tender. Toss potatoes with lime juice and remaining ¼ teaspoon salt.

2. While potatoes roast, stir together ketchup, ginger, curry powder, and cayenne in a small bowl. Serve fries with ketchup.

Serving size: About 8 fries and 2 tablespoons ketchup
Calories 131; Fat 3.7g (sat 0.5g, mono 2.5g, poly 0.5g); Cholesterol 0mg; Protein 2g; Carbohydrate 24g; Sugars 12g; Fiber 3g; RS 1g; Sodium 599mg

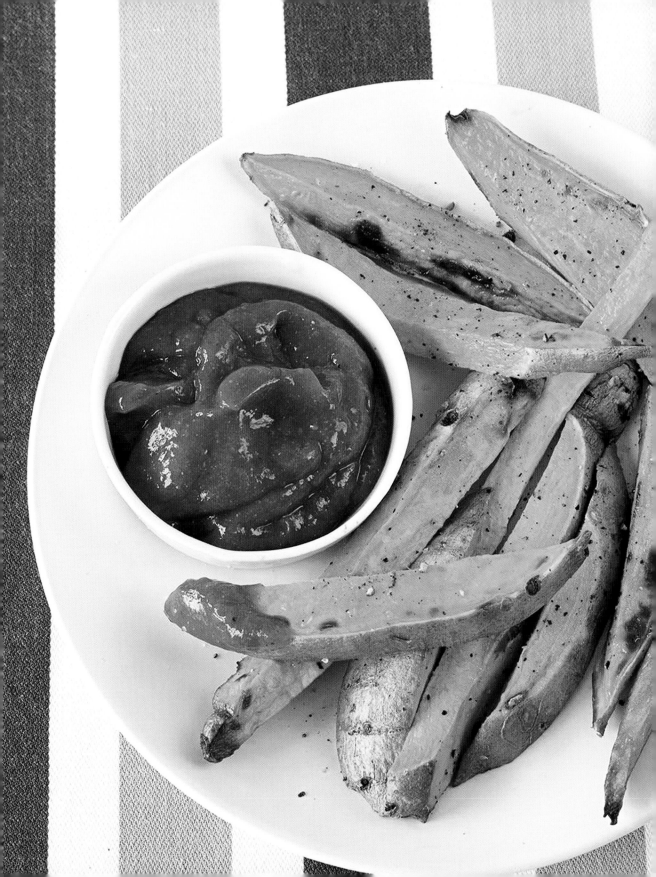

RS
1.9g

Potato Gratin Casserole

Prep: *10 minutes* | ***Cook:*** *25 minutes* | ***Total time:*** *35 minutes* | ***Makes:*** *8 servings*

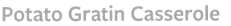

Want to bring a Resistant Starch–filled dish to your next potluck or family gathering? This rustic casserole is super satisfying and an absolute crowd-pleaser.

3 pounds red potatoes, scrubbed and quartered
4 sprigs thyme plus 1 tablespoon thyme leaves, divided
1 garlic clove, peeled
¾ cup low-fat (2%) milk
2 tablespoons unsalted butter
½ cup grated Parmesan cheese (2 ounces), divided
⅛ teaspoon salt
¼ teaspoon pepper
½ cup panko (Japanese bread crumbs)

1. Place potatoes, thyme sprigs, and garlic in a large saucepan and cover with cold water. Bring to a boil over high heat. Reduce heat; simmer, uncovered, about 20 minutes, until potatoes are tender (test with a knife). Reserve ½ cup cooking water; drain. Return potatoes to pot over low heat.

2. Add milk, reserved cooking water, butter, ¼ cup Parmesan, salt, and pepper. Mash potatoes with a large fork or potato masher until smooth. Transfer potatoes to a shallow 1½-quart ovenproof casserole or baking dish.

3. Preheat broiler. Combine panko, remaining ¼ cup Parmesan, and thyme leaves; sprinkle over potatoes. Broil 4–5 inches from heat source until cheese melts and starts to brown, 3–4 minutes. Serve warm.

Serving size: 1 cup Calories 204; Fat 4.9g (sat 3g, mono 1.3g, poly 0.2g); Cholesterol 14mg; Protein 6g; Carbohydrate 35g; Sugars 3g; Fiber 3g; RS 1.9g; Sodium 138mg

TIP:
If you're bringing this to someone's house, make the casserole through step 2. Finish it under the broiler before dinner is served.

German Potato Salad

RS
0.8g

Prep: 15 minutes | **Cook:** 30 minutes | **Total time:** 45 minutes | **Makes:** 12 servings

Tangy and just a bit sweet, this potato salad is a bacon lover's dream. It's yummy served warm or cold and is always a hit at summer picnics and barbecues.

2 pounds russet potatoes
3 tablespoons olive oil, divided
4 ounces turkey bacon, diced
2 ribs celery, thinly sliced (⅔ cup)
⅔ cup finely minced onion
½ cup apple cider vinegar
2 tablespoons whole grain Dijon mustard
1 tablespoon sugar
½ teaspoon salt
½ teaspoon pepper
½ cup chopped dill pickle (3-ounce pickle)
3 hard-boiled eggs, chopped
3 tablespoons chopped fresh dill

1. Place potatoes in a saucepan and cover with cold water. Bring to a boil, reduce heat, and cook until potatoes are fork-tender but not mushy, 20 minutes. Drain, cool, cut into 1-inch cubes, and place in a large bowl.

2. Heat 1 tablespoon oil in a large nonstick skillet over medium-high heat. Add bacon and cook until crisp, 4–5 minutes. Carefully remove bacon from skillet, reserving oil; drain bacon on paper towels. Add celery and onion to oil and cook until just softened, 2 minutes. Whisk together vinegar, ½ cup water, mustard, sugar, salt, pepper, and remaining 2 tablespoons oil; add to skillet.

3. Bring to a boil, reduce heat, and simmer until partially reduced, 2 minutes. Pour over potatoes and add bacon, pickle, eggs, and dill. Toss to fold gently. Chill or serve at room temperature.

Serving size: ½ cup Calories 157; Fat 6.6g (sat 1.4g, mono 3.6g, poly 1.1g); Cholesterol 55mg; Protein 5g; Carbohydrate 19g; Sugars 3g; Fiber 2g; RS 0.8g; Sodium 353mg

RS
1.9g

Herb and Olive Oil Mashed Potatoes

Prep: 5 minutes | *Cook:* 20 minutes | *Total time:* 25 minutes | *Makes:* 4 servings

Mashed potatoes are a welcome sight on any dinner table. Our version gets extra flavor from cooking the potatoes with garlic, and then mashing them with thyme.

1½ pounds red potatoes, scrubbed and cubed
3 garlic cloves, peeled and thinly sliced
3 tablespoons olive oil
1 tablespoon thyme leaves
½ teaspoon salt
¼ teaspoon pepper
1 tablespoon chopped parsley

1. Place potatoes and garlic in a large saucepan and cover with cold water. Bring to a boil over high heat. Reduce heat; simmer, uncovered, about 20 minutes, until potatoes are tender (test with a knife). Reserve ½ cup cooking water; drain. Return potatoes to pot over low heat.

2. Meanwhile, heat oil and thyme in a small skillet over medium heat. Cook until thyme sizzles, about 2 minutes.

3. Add ¼ cup of the reserved cooking water, oil with thyme, salt, and pepper to potatoes. Mash with a potato masher to desired consistency (add more cooking water if necessary). Stir in parsley.

Serving size: 1¼ cups Calories 221; Fat 10.3g (sat 1.4g, mono 7.4g, poly 1.1g); Cholesterol 0mg; Protein 3g; Carbohydrate 30g; Sugars 1g; Fiber 3g; RS 1.9g; Sodium 298mg

Savory Cornbread Stuffing

Prep: 10 minutes | **Cook:** 60 minutes | **Total time:** 70 minutes | **Makes:** 4 servings

Warm and comforting, this stuffing is perfect. We love it with our Thanksgiving turkey, but it's a wonderful side dish with any fall or winter meal.

4	cups cornbread, cut into 1-inch cubes
2	teaspoons olive oil
1	medium onion, chopped
2	cloves garlic, minced
1	tablespoon dried rubbed sage
2	ribs celery, chopped
1	small apple, diced (1 cup)
⅓	cup dried cranberries
1½	cups low-sodium chicken stock
1	egg
	Cooking spray

1. Preheat oven to 350°. Place cornbread on a baking sheet and toast lightly, 8–10 minutes. Remove from oven and cool.

2. Heat oil in a large high-sided skillet; add onion and cook, stirring occasionally, until lightly browned, 8–9 minutes. Add garlic and sage and cook 1 minute. Add celery and apple and cook until crisp-tender, 2–3 minutes.

3. Add toasted stuffing and cranberries and stir gently to combine. Remove pan from heat and cool slightly.

4. Whisk together stock and egg; add to cornbread mixture. Gently stir until moistened. Coat an 8-inch baking dish with cooking spray and transfer mixture to dish. Bake until top is browned, 35–40 minutes.

Serving size: ¾ cup stuffing Calories 270; Fat 8.5g (sat 1.7g, mono 3.7g, poly 2.5g); Cholesterol 69mg; Protein 7g; Carbohydrate 43g; Sugars 12g; Fiber 4g; RS 0g; Sodium 436mg

TIP:
Save time and pick up store-bought cornbread instead of making your own. Or make one, cube it, and freeze it before the holidays!

RS
0.7g

Honey-Glazed Roasted Root Vegetables

Prep: 15 minutes | **Cook:** 50 minutes | **Total time:** 1 hour 5 minutes | **Makes:** 6 servings

The earthy flavors of fall come together in this warming dish. It's a wonderful accompaniment to roast chicken or pork.

2 tablespoons olive oil
2 tablespoons honey
1 teaspoon salt
¼ teaspoon pepper
2 teaspoons chopped fresh
   rosemary
1 pound carrots (about 6 large),
   peeled and cut into 2-inch chunks
1 pound parsnips (about 1 large),
   peeled and cut into 2-inch chunks
1 pound yams (about 2 medium),
   skin-on, cut into 2-inch chunks
1 large red onion, peeled and cut
   into 1-inch wedges
15 cloves peeled garlic

1. Preheat oven to 425°.

2. Whisk together oil, honey, salt, pepper, and rosemary in a large bowl; add remaining ingredients and toss. Spread on a foil-lined baking sheet. Roast for 30 minutes until underside of vegetables is golden brown. Remove from oven. Using a spatula, turn vegetables and return to oven until golden brown and cooked through but not mushy, 20–30 minutes. Serve hot or at room temperature.

Serving size: 1 cup Calories 215; Fat 5.1g (sat 0.7g, mono 3.4g, poly 0.7g); Cholesterol 0mg; Protein 3g; Carbohydrate 42g; Sugars 17g; Fiber 8g; RS 0.7g; Sodium 466mg

TIP:
If you have leftover roasted vegetables, you can use them to make a quick soup, or purée them in a food processor with a little olive oil for a delicious dip.

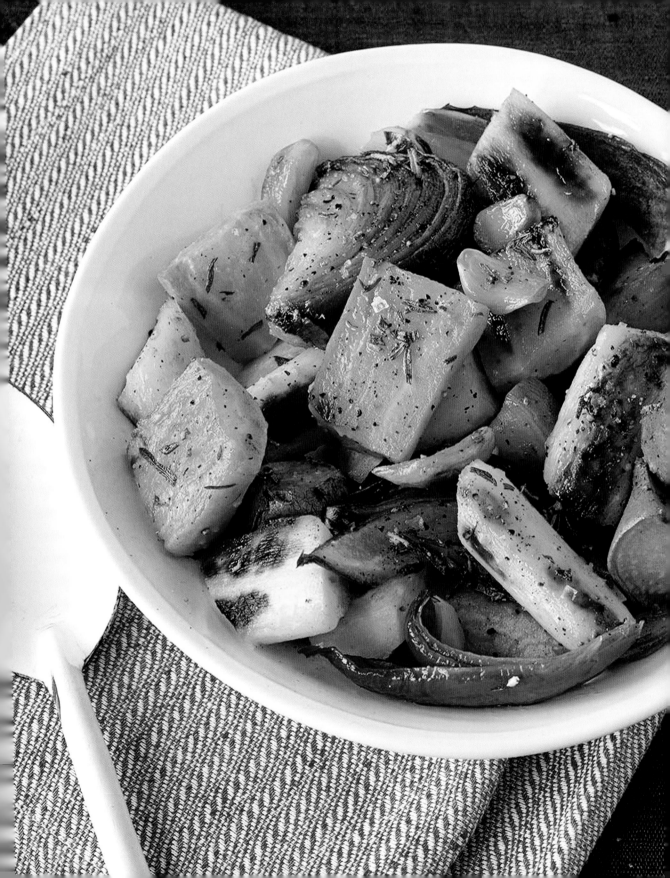

Crispy Onion Rings

Prep: *10 minutes* | **Cook:** *15 minutes* | **Total time:** *25 minutes* | **Makes:** *4 servings*

This bar-food favorite was begging for a CarbLovers makeover! Using cornflakes adds Resistant Starch, and baking instead of deep-frying helps slash the calories and fat.

2 cups cornflakes
20 saltines, coarsely crushed
1½ teaspoons olive oil
¼ teaspoon kosher salt
¼ teaspoon freshly ground black pepper
1 large egg white
½ cup all-purpose flour
½ teaspoon paprika
½ cup low-fat buttermilk
Cooking spray
1 large sweet onion (about 1½ pounds), cut into ¾-inch slices

1. Preheat oven to 450°. Combine cornflakes and saltines in a food processor; pulse until fine crumbs form (1½ cups). Add oil; pulse to distribute. Add salt and pepper; pulse. Transfer crumbs to a shallow dish. Whisk together egg white, flour, paprika, buttermilk, and 2 tablespoons water in a medium bowl.

2. Coat 2 large rimmed baking sheets with cooking spray; transfer to oven to heat, 2 minutes. Separate onion slices into individual rings. Dip onion rings in batter, then crumb mixture; carefully transfer to hot baking sheets and arrange in a single layer. Bake, turning once, until onion rings are golden brown, about 15 minutes. Serve hot.

Serving size: 3–4 onion rings Calories 279; Fat 5.8g (sat 1.1g, mono 3.2g, poly 1.2g); Cholesterol 1mg; Protein 7g; Carbohydrate 50g; Sugars 12g; Fiber 3g; RS 0.5g; Sodium 450mg

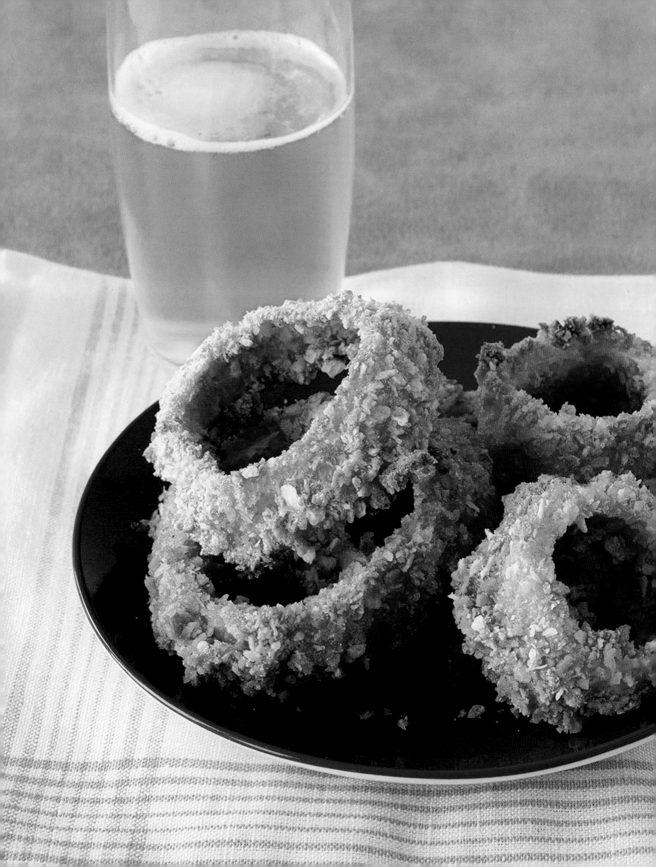

Fried Brown Rice with Edamame

Prep: 1 minute | Cook: 4 minutes | Total time: 5 minutes | Makes: 4 servings

No time to cook? As long as you have frozen or microwaveable rice on hand, this dish comes together in minutes.

- 2 tablespoons vegetable oil
- 2 cups cooked brown rice (such as Uncle Ben's Ready Rice; use an 8.8-ounce bag)
- 2 large eggs, lightly beaten
- 2 cups coleslaw mix
- 1 cup frozen shelled edamame, thawed
- 2 tablespoons reduced-sodium soy sauce
- 1 tablespoon chile-garlic sauce (such as Sriracha)
- ¼ cup cilantro leaves
- ¼ cup peanuts, chopped

Heat oil in a large heavy-bottomed skillet over high heat. Add rice; cook until heated through, about 1 minute. Stir eggs into rice; cook 30 seconds. Stir in coleslaw mix, edamame, soy sauce, and chile-garlic sauce; cook 2 minutes or until eggs are cooked and edamame are heated through. Serve rice topped with cilantro and peanuts.

Serving size: 1 cup fried rice Calories 318; Fat 16.3g (sat 2.1g, mono 5g, poly 6.6g); Cholesterol 93mg; Protein 14g; Carbohydrate 30g; Sugars 4g; Fiber 5g; RS 1.7g; Sodium 429mg

TIP:
Great for flexitarians! Add a handful of sautéed shrimp to boost the protein in this quick dish.

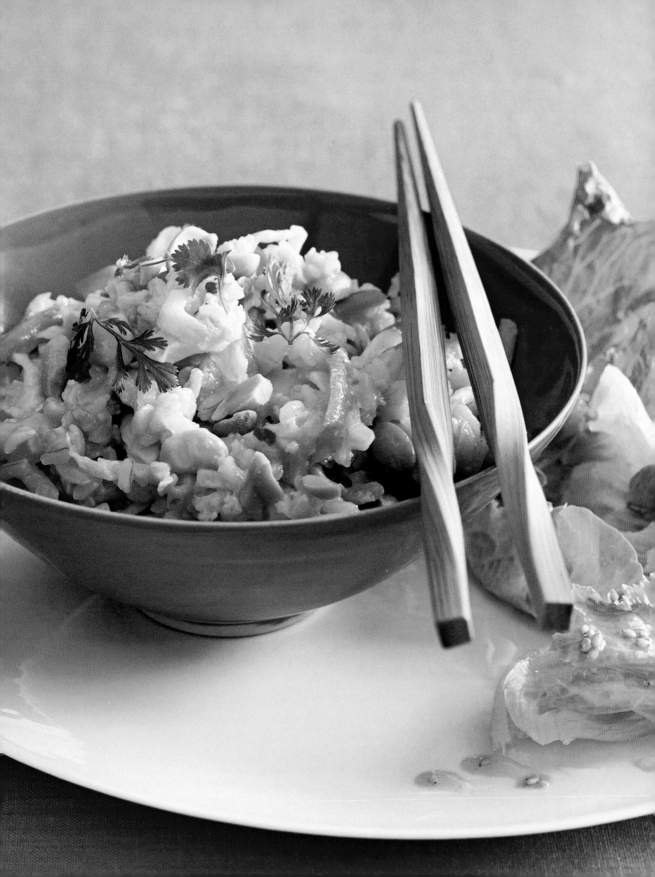

RS
3.1g

Hoppin' John

Prep: *10 minutes* | **Cook:** *20 minutes* | **Total time:** *30 minutes* | **Makes:** *4 servings*

Tradition says that if you start the New Year with a bowl of Hoppin' John, you'll have good luck all year long. All we know for sure is that this dish is a super tasty way to get your Resistant Starch!

2 ounces sliced pancetta, chopped
1 shallot, finely chopped
1 bunch collard greens, chopped (about 10 cups), thick stems discarded
1 cup low-sodium chicken broth
1 tablespoon cider vinegar
1 (14.5-ounce) can diced tomatoes
¼ teaspoon crushed red pepper
1 (15-ounce) can black-eyed peas, rinsed and drained
4 cups cooked brown rice, warmed

1. Heat a large high-sided skillet over medium heat. Add pancetta; cook, stirring, until browned and crisp, 4 to 6 minutes. Transfer pancetta with a slotted spoon to a paper towel–lined plate to drain; reserve fat in skillet. Add shallot; cook over medium-high heat, stirring occasionally, until tender and golden, about 3 minutes.

2. Add collard greens, broth, vinegar, tomatoes, and crushed red pepper; bring to a boil. Simmer, covered, 5 minutes; stir in black-eyed peas. Cook 5 minutes or until greens and black-eyed peas are tender.

3. Serve greens and black-eyed peas over rice; sprinkle with reserved pancetta.

Serving size: 1¼ cups Calories 364; Fat 6.9g (sat 2.5g, mono 2.6g, poly 1.9g); Cholesterol 10mg; Protein 15g; Carbohydrate 62g; Sugars 7g; Fiber 12g; RS 3.1g; Sodium 618mg

RS
1.4g

Wild Rice Pilaf with Pecans, Cranberries, and Scallions

Prep: 10 minutes | **Cook:** 45 minutes | **Total time:** 55 minutes | **Makes:** 12 servings

This delicious dish has a wonderful blend of nutty rice, chewy cranberries, and crunchy pecans. It makes a pretty addition to any holiday feast.

1 tablespoon olive oil
1 medium onion, chopped
1 teaspoon minced garlic
2½ cups wild- and brown-rice mix (such as Lundberg Wild Blend), cooked according to package instructions (about 6 cups cooked)
⅓ cup dried cranberries
¼ cup toasted chopped pecans
½ cup chopped scallions
¾ teaspoon salt
½ teaspoon pepper

1. Heat oil in a large saucepan over medium-high heat. Add onion and cook, stirring occasionally, until tender and golden, 8–9 minutes. Add garlic and cook 1 minute.

2. Add rice and cook until heated through, 1–2 minutes. Transfer to serving dish and toss with cranberries, pecans, scallions, salt, and pepper. Serve warm.

Serving size: ½ cup Calories 181; Fat 3.7g (sat 0.5g, mono 2g, poly 1g); Cholesterol 0mg; Protein 5g; Carbohydrate 33g; Sugars 3g; Fiber 3g; RS 1.4g; Sodium 152mg

TIP:
Try swapping out the cranberries for dried cherries, and experiment with different nuts.

Appetizers & Cocktails

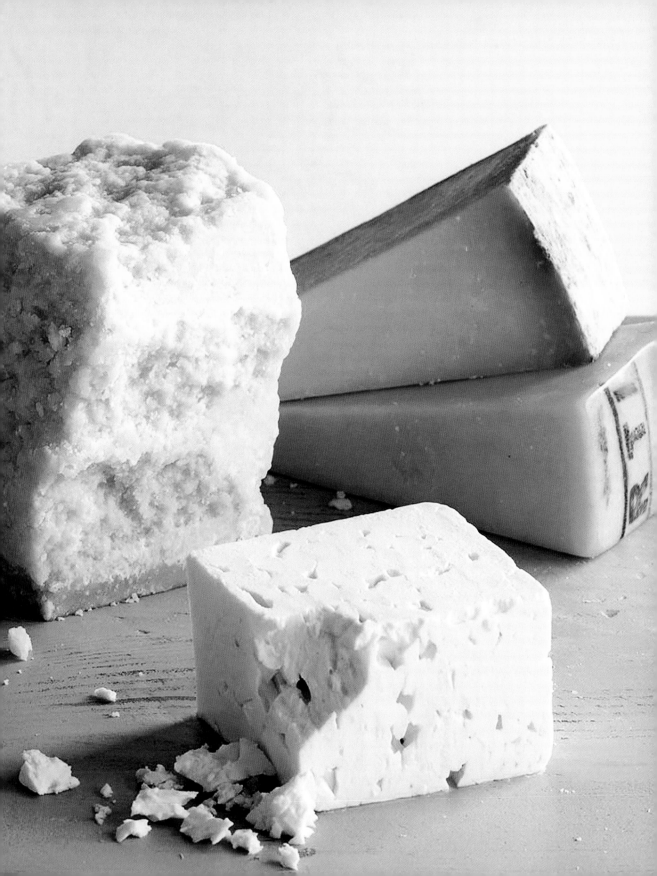

Ham and Cheddar Potato Skins

Prep: *10 minutes* | **Cook:** *30 minutes* | **Total time:** *40 minutes* | **Makes:** *6 servings*

We took this traditionally high-fat nibble and gave it a CarbLovers *makeover. Using smaller potatoes keeps these bites portion-controlled.*

6   small potatoes (1½ pounds)
2   tablespoons reduced-fat sour
     cream
¼   teaspoon kosher salt
¼   teaspoon freshly ground black
     pepper
2   scallions, sliced (white and green
     parts separated)
2   ounces sliced deli ham, chopped
½   cup grated sharp cheddar cheese

1. Preheat oven to 350°.

2. Bake potatoes on baking sheet 25–30 minutes or until tender; set aside to cool. Preheat broiler with rack in highest position.

3. Halve cooked potatoes lengthwise. Scoop out flesh, leaving a ¼-inch border; transfer potato flesh (about 2 cups) to a bowl. Mash potato with sour cream and 2 tablespoons water; season with salt and pepper. Fold in scallion whites and ham; spoon filling into potato shells.

4. Arrange filled potato skins on a baking sheet; sprinkle evenly with cheese. Broil 5 minutes or until cheese is melted. Sprinkle with scallion greens before serving, if desired.

Serving size: 2 potato skins Calories 186; Fat 4.3g (sat 2.5g, mono 1.2g, poly 0.2g); Cholesterol 16mg; Protein 7g; Carbohydrate 30g; Sugars 2g; Fiber 3g; RS 1.4g; Sodium 279mg

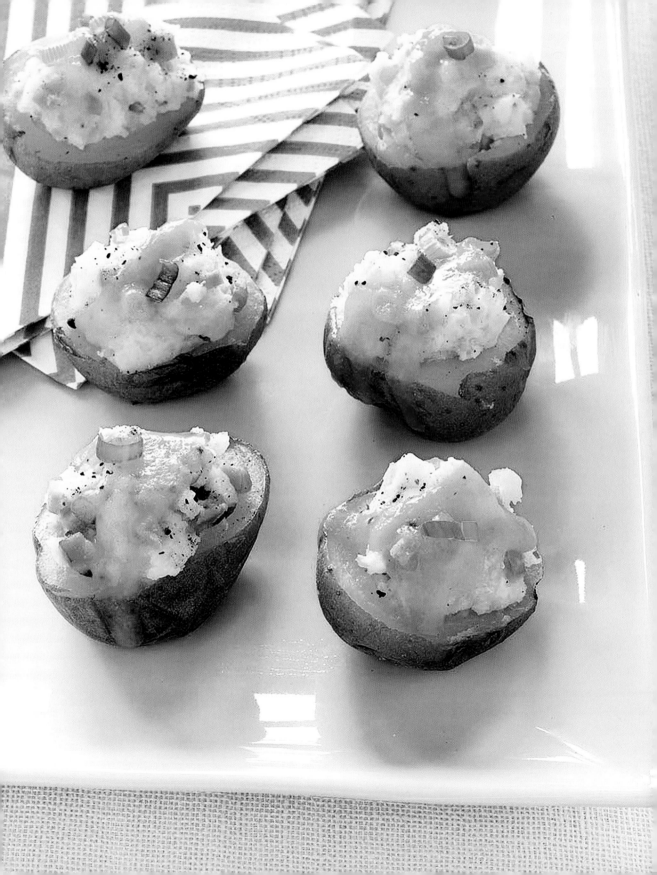

RS
0.7g

Layered Spicy Black Bean and Cheddar Dip

Prep: 20 minutes | **Total time:** 20 minutes | **Makes:** 8 servings

This is the ultimate "wow" party dip, especially for game day! It's super-flavorful, filling, and makes for a stunning presentation.

1   medium avocado, pitted
    (about 1 cup mashed)
1   tablespoon fresh lime juice
1   teaspoon lime zest
¼   teaspoon salt, divided
¼   teaspoon pepper, divided
1   (15-ounce) can low-sodium black
    beans, rinsed and drained
1   teaspoon Tabasco
⅓   cup chopped red onion, divided
1   cup jarred salsa
1   cup reduced-fat sour cream
¼   cup chopped tomato
¼   cup chopped scallions
    Large bag of tortilla chips for
    serving (such as Food Should
    Taste Good)

1. Mash avocado, lime juice, lime zest, and half of the salt and pepper in a bowl; set aside.

2. Mash beans, Tabasco, and remaining salt and pepper in another bowl.

3. Place black bean mixture on the bottom of a 4-cup crock or glass bowl. Layer avocado mash on top of beans, then sprinkle with ¼ cup of the red onion. Top with salsa, then with sour cream. Top with chopped tomato, scallions, and remaining red onion.

4. Serve dip with tortilla chips.

Serving size: ½ cup dip and 5 chips Calories 199; Fat 9.6g (sat 2.9g, mono 4.9g, poly 1.1g); Cholesterol 12mg; Protein 6g; Carbohydrate 23g; Sugars 2g; Fiber 6g; RS 0.7g; Sodium 345mg

ASK CARBLOVERS

Q: What can I drink (besides plain water) when I'm out with friends?

A: Unsweetened tea, coffee (iced or hot), and water spiked with citrus fruit or cucumber slices can be enjoyed anytime. After the Kickstart, you can have a 5-ounce glass of wine or 12-ounce bottle of light beer as one of your daily snacks.

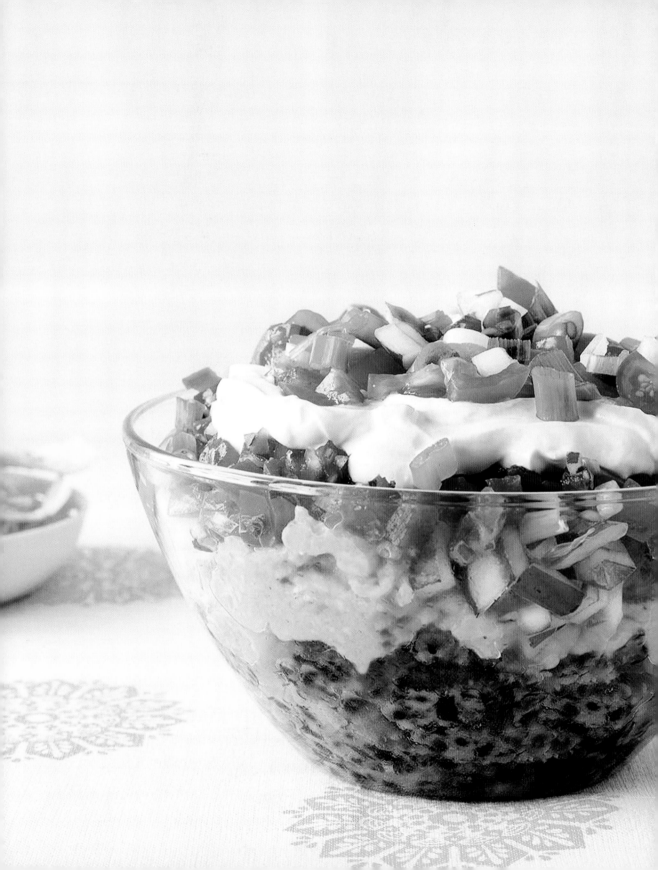

RS
1.4g

Pumpernickel Toasts with Smoked Salmon and Lemon-Chive Cream

Prep: *10 minutes* | **Total time:** *10 minutes* | **Makes:** *6 servings*

The classic combination of pumpernickel and smoked salmon gets livened up with a dollop of our tangy lemon cream.

½ cup 2% Greek yogurt

2 tablespoons chopped fresh chives, plus more for garnish

1 tablespoon olive oil

½ teaspoon finely grated lemon zest

2 ounces smoked salmon

18 small pumpernickel toasts

1. Stir together yogurt, chives, oil, and zest in a small bowl.

2. Divide salmon among pumpernickel toasts; top each with about 1½ teaspoons yogurt mixture. Sprinkle with remaining chives and serve.

Serving size: 3 toasts Calories 119; Fat 4g (sat 0.8g, mono 2.1g, poly 0.7g); Cholesterol 3mg; Protein 6g; Carbohydrate 15g; Sugars 1g; Fiber 2g; RS 1.4g; Sodium 282mg

TIP:
Serve these bites for brunch with a crisp sparkling wine or the *CarbLovers* Fat-Flushing Cocktail, page 28.

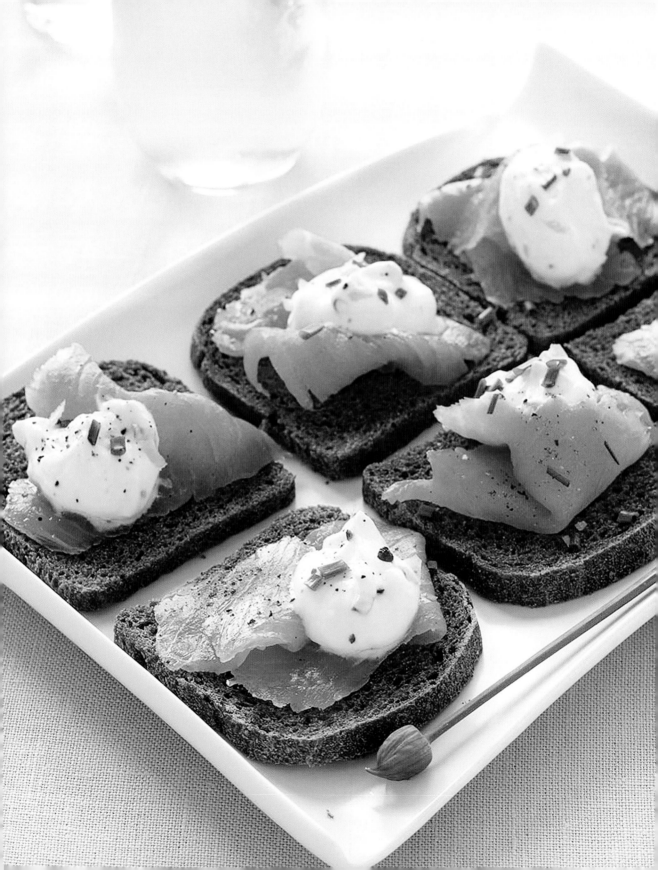

Mini Corn and Feta Muffins

Prep: *5 minutes* | **Cook:** *15 minutes* | **Total time:** *20 minutes* | **Makes:** *10 servings*

These savory muffins get a flavor kick from feta cheese and buttermilk. They're easy to whip up on a weeknight and go perfectly with our Mexican Mole Chile on page 84.

½ cup all-purpose flour
½ cup cornmeal
1 tablespoon sugar
1 teaspoon baking powder
¼ teaspoon salt
¼ teaspoon ground pepper
⅓ cup buttermilk
2 tablespoons melted butter
1 large egg white
⅓ cup crumbled feta cheese
½ cup thawed corn kernels
Cooking spray

1. Preheat oven to 425°.

2. Whisk together flour, cornmeal, sugar, baking powder, salt, and pepper in a medium bowl; make a well in center of mixture. Combine buttermilk, butter, and egg white in a small bowl; add to flour mixture, stirring until just moist. Fold in feta and corn.

3. Coat a 20-cup mini muffin pan with cooking spray. Spoon batter into prepared pan; bake for 10–12 minutes or until muffins spring back when touched lightly in center. Remove muffins from pan immediately; place on a wire rack. Serve warm.

Serving size: 2 muffins Calories 107; Fat 4g (sat 2.4g, mono 1.2g, poly 0.3g); Cholesterol 11mg; Protein 3g; Carbohydrate 15g; Sugars 2g; Fiber 1g; RS 0g; Sodium 178mg

> **TIP:**
> Make a double batch of these muffins, cool, and freeze in a resealable bag. Then, pop them in the microwave for 20–30 seconds before serving.

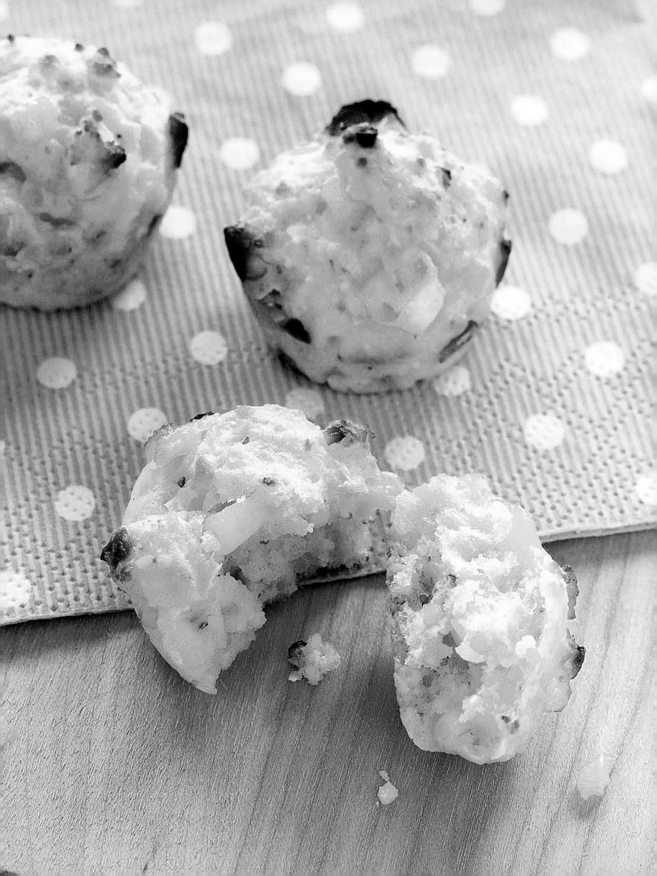

RS
1g

Smoky Oven-Baked Potato Chips

Prep: *15 minutes* | **Cook:** *25 minutes* | **Total time:** *40 minutes* | **Makes:** *About 6 servings*

Potato chips are back on the menu! These are lighter than most store-bought varieties because we oven-bake them. Smoked paprika makes them even more flavorful.

2 russet potatoes (about 1½ pounds), scrubbed
2 tablespoons olive oil
1 teaspoon smoked paprika
¾ teaspoon salt, divided
¼ teaspoon pepper

1. Preheat oven to 400°.

2. Using a mandolin slicer or sharp knife, slice potatoes into ⅛-inch-thick rounds. Pat dry on layers of paper towels to absorb as much moisture as possible.

3. Toss potato slices with oil in a large bowl, then toss with smoked paprika, ½ teaspoon salt, and pepper; arrange in a single layer on baking sheets.

4. Bake until browned and potato edges lift slightly from baking sheets, 20–25 minutes. Remove from oven and sprinkle with remaining ¼ teaspoon salt.

5. Cool completely and store in an airtight container for up to 1 day.

Serving size: About 11 chips Calories 130; Fat 4.7g (sat 0.7g, mono 3.3g, poly 0.5g); Cholesterol 0mg; Protein 2g; Carbohydrate 20g; Sugars 1g; Fiber 2g; RS 1g; Sodium 298mg

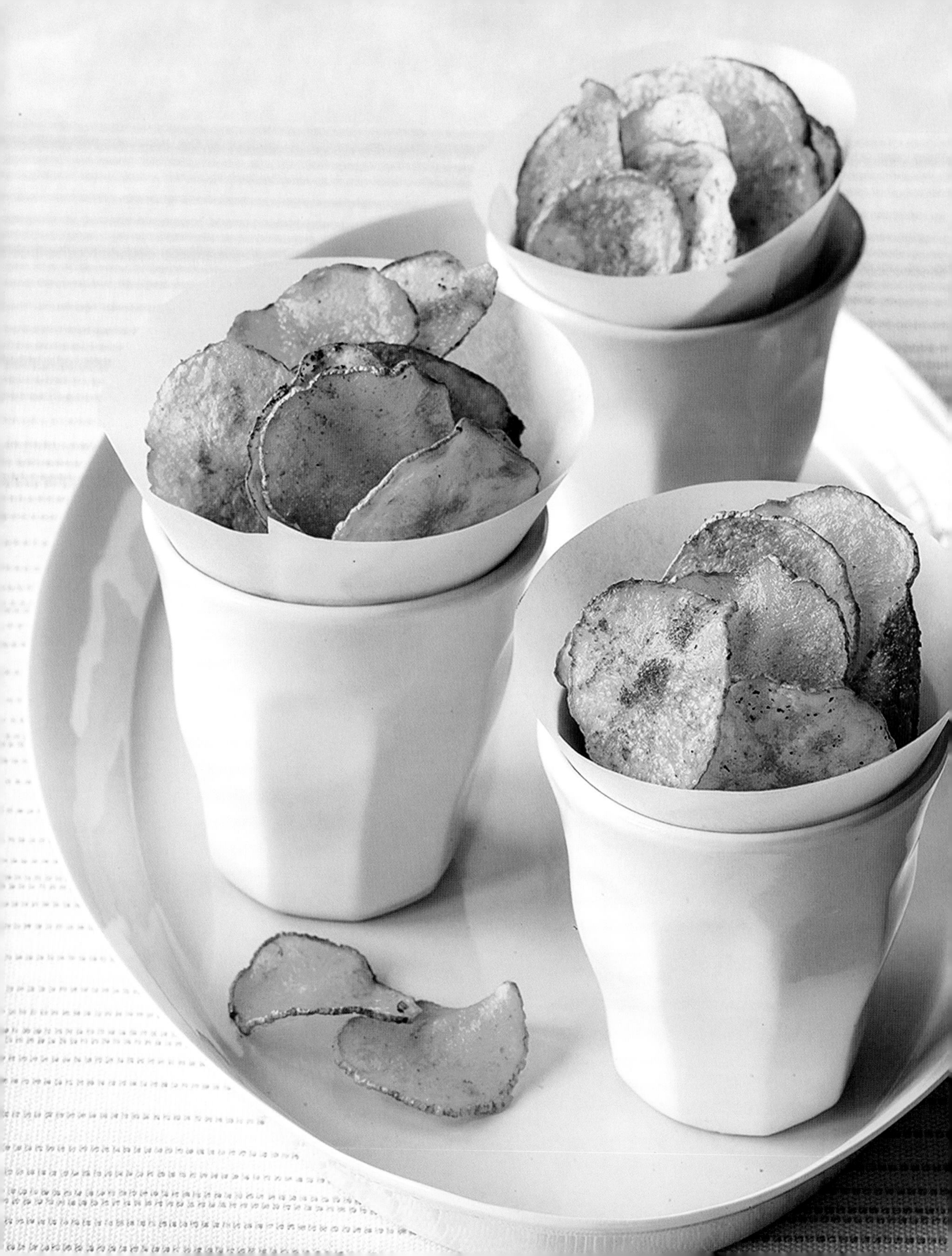

RS
0.5g

Edamame and Mushroom Potstickers

Prep: *35 minutes* | **Cook:** *10 minutes* | **Total time:** *45 minutes* | **Makes:** *6 servings*

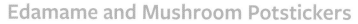

Savory and fun to eat, these bites make a perfect prelude to an Asian-themed meal.

1 tablespoon vegetable oil, divided
2 scallions, greens sliced and whites finely chopped
1 tablespoon finely chopped ginger
2 garlic cloves, finely chopped
6 ounces shiitake mushrooms, halved
⅓ cup frozen shelled edamame, thawed
¼ cup low-sodium soy sauce, divided
2 teaspoons sesame oil
1 large egg white
¼ teaspoon kosher salt
¼ teaspoon freshly ground pepper
18 (2- to 3-inch square) wontons (from a 12-ounce package), such as Nasoya brand

1. Heat 1 teaspoon vegetable oil in a large nonstick skillet over medium heat. Add scallion whites, ginger, and garlic to skillet; cook until fragrant, 1 minute. Add mushrooms to skillet; cook, tossing occasionally, until browned, about 5 minutes. Transfer mushrooms to a food processor with edamame, 1 tablespoon soy sauce, and sesame oil; pulse until finely chopped. Add egg white, salt, and pepper; pulse to combine. (Wipe out skillet and reserve.)

2. Arrange wontons. Use a dampened finger to trace around wonton edge; place about 2 teaspoons filling in each. Fold wonton over to cover filling; press to seal edge. Transfer dumplings to a plate; cover with a damp paper towel until needed.

3. Heat 1 teaspoon oil in reserved skillet over medium heat. Add half of wontons to skillet; cook 2 minutes or until browned on one side. Add ¼ cup water to pan; cover and cook until cooked through, 3–4 minutes. Cook second batch of wontons in remaining 1 teaspoon of oil. Serve with remaining scallion greens and soy sauce.

Serving size: 3 potstickers Calories 116; Fat 4.5g (sat 0.4g, mono 1.2g, poly 2.2g); Cholesterol 3mg; Protein 5g; Carbohydrate 14g; Sugars 1g; Fiber 2g; RS 0.5g; Sodium 608mg

TIP:
To store, freeze wontons on a wax paper–lined plate until firm and store in a resealable freezer bag for up to 3 months.

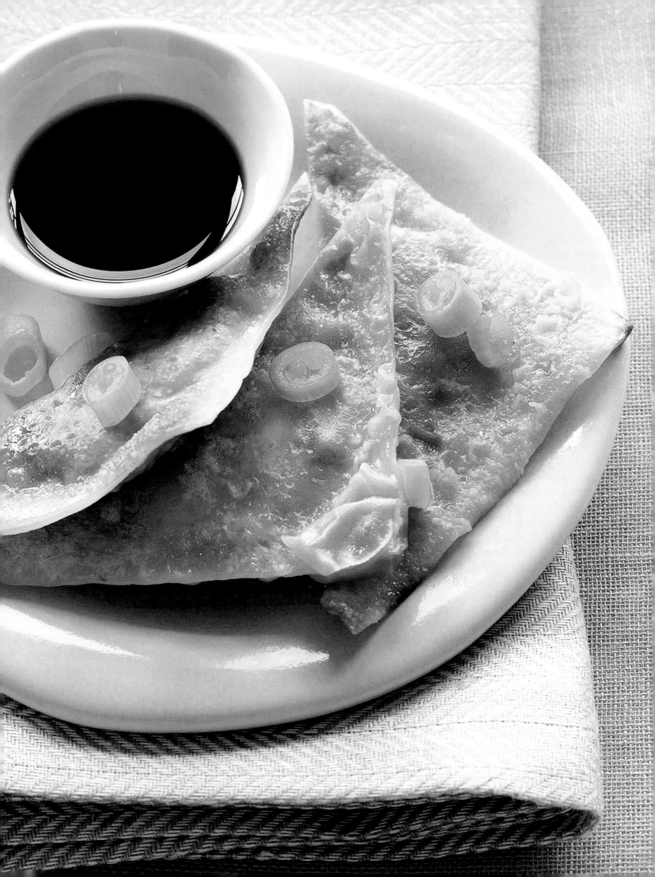

Garbanzo Bean and Artichoke Bruschetta

Prep: *5 minutes* | **Cook:** *20 minutes* | **Total time:** *25 minutes* | **Makes:** *6 servings*

Quick and versatile, bruschetta is one of our favorite appetizers to make. This one is packed with fiber and absolutely delicious.

½ (5 ounces total) baguette, sliced into ⅛-inch rounds
1 (13.75-ounce) can artichokes in water, drained and chopped
1 (15-ounce) can garbanzo beans, rinsed and drained
2 tablespoons olive oil
1 tablespoon fresh lemon juice
1 tablespoon chopped parsley
¼ teaspoon salt
¼ teaspoon pepper
1 garlic clove, peeled and halved

1. Preheat oven to 350°. Arrange baguette slices in a single layer on baking sheet; bake about 20 minutes or until crispy. Set aside to cool completely.

2. Meanwhile, stir together artichokes, beans, oil, lemon juice, parsley, salt, and pepper.

3. Rub tops of toasted bread slices with cut side of garlic; top with bean mixture and serve.

Serving size: About 4 bruschetta Calories 220; Fat 5.5g (sat 0.7g, mono 3.4g, poly 0.7g); Cholesterol 0mg; Protein 9g; Carbohydrate 34g; Sugars 1g; Fiber 6g; RS 0.5g; Sodium 631mg

RS
0.7g

Cinnamon-Sugar Tortilla Chips

Prep: *5 minutes* | **Cook:** *10 minutes* | **Total time:** *15 minutes* | **Makes:** *4 servings*

We love making homemade chips from tortillas, and this sweet spin is a fun changeup from the usual savory ones.

4 (6-inch) corn tortillas
1 tablespoon vegetable oil
1 tablespoon sugar
½ teaspoon ground cinnamon
⅛ teaspoon salt

1. Preheat oven to 400°.

2. Brush both sides of tortillas with oil. Using a pizza cutter or clean kitchen shears, cut each tortilla into 8 equal-size triangles.

3. Combine sugar, cinnamon, and salt in a large bowl. Add tortilla crisps and toss to coat.

4. Place on a baking sheet and bake until crisp, 10–12 minutes. Remove, cool, and serve.

Serving size: 8 chips Calories 101; Fat 4g (sat 0.3g, mono 0.9g, poly 2.5g); Cholesterol 0mg; Protein 1g; Carbohydrate 16g; Sugars 3g; Fiber 2g; RS 0.7g; Sodium 76mg

TIP:
If you're looking for a dip to serve these with, just combine 1 cup low-fat vanilla yogurt with 2 teaspoons honey.

RS
0.2g

Roasted Red Pepper and Zucchini Spread

Prep: *10 minutes* | **Cook:** *10 minutes* | **Total time:** *20 minutes* | **Makes:** *8 servings*

Zesty and bold, this richly textured spread is fabulous for parties, and also helps jazz up sandwiches and wraps.

1   large (1-pound) zucchini, sliced into ½-inch rings
1   (15-ounce) jar roasted red peppers, rinsed, drained, and patted dry
2   tablespoons olive oil
4   teaspoons red wine vinegar
3   tablespoons chopped parsley
2   teaspoons minced garlic
2   ounces crumbled feta cheese
½   teaspoon black pepper
1   (10-ounce) baguette, sliced into ¼-inch rounds and toasted

1. Preheat broiler. Arrange zucchini slices in a single layer on a baking sheet and broil until tops are well charred and slices are slightly wilted, about 10 minutes.

2. Remove from oven and cool for 10 minutes.

3. Place cooled zucchini, peppers, oil, vinegar, parsley, garlic, feta, and pepper in a food processor and pulse until incorporated but still chunky, 15–20 pulses.

4. Serve spread on toasted baguette slices.

Serving size: ¼ cup dip plus 3 baguette slices Calories 94; Fat 5.4g (sat 1.6g, mono 2.8g, poly 0.6g); Cholesterol 6mg; Protein 3g; Carbohydrate 9g; Sugars 3g; Fiber 1g; RS 0.2g; Sodium 268mg

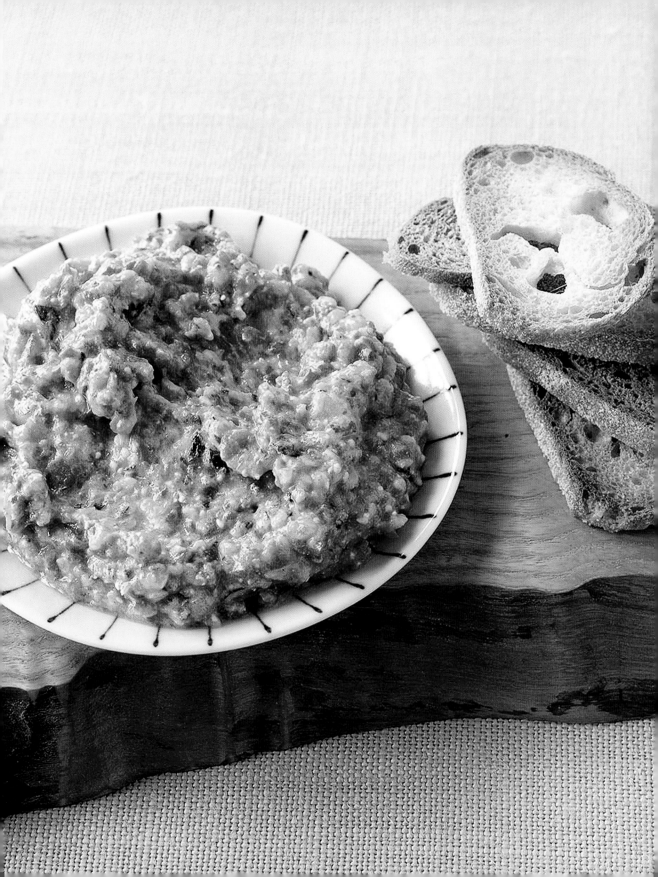

RS 0.5g

Creamy Spinach-Artichoke Dip

Prep: *5 minutes* | ***Cook:*** *5 minutes* | ***Total time:*** *10 minutes* | ***Makes:*** *8 servings*

This all-time favorite dip is typically packed with sodium and saturated fat. Our delicious version adds in Resistant Starch and slashes the salt and fat.

1 (12-ounce) jar water-packed artichokes, drained well and patted dry

1 (10-ounce) package frozen spinach, thawed and water squeezed out

4 tablespoons light mayonnaise

4 tablespoons reduced-fat mayonnaise

½ cup canned low-sodium white beans, rinsed and drained

½ ounce (½ cup) freshly grated Parmesan cheese

2 tablespoons water

2 teaspoons minced garlic

¼ teaspoon salt

½ teaspoon pepper

4 cups assorted raw vegetables, such as broccoli, zucchini, and sugar snap peas

1. Combine all ingredients in a food processor and blend until smooth, 20 seconds. Serve with veggies or chips.

Serving size: ¼ cup dip and ½ cup assorted raw veggies
Calories 109; Fat 4.3g (sat 1g, mono 0.8g, poly 1.5g); Cholesterol 4mg; Protein 6g; Carbohydrate 14g; Sugars 2g; Fiber 4g; RS 0.5g; Sodium 528mg

Rosemary and Garlic White Bean Dip

Prep: *5 minutes* | **Cook:** *2 minutes* | **Total time:** *7 minutes* | **Makes:** *12 servings*

This creamy Tuscan dip and chip combo packs 2 grams of Resistant Starch into just 225 calories. Try the dip with chopped veggies too!

2 tablespoons olive oil, plus more for serving

4 garlic cloves, sliced

2 tablespoon fresh rosemary leaves, plus more for garnish

2 (15-ounce) cans cannellini beans, rinsed and drained

2 tablespoons fresh lemon juice

10 ounces pita chips, for serving

1. Heat oil in a small skillet over medium heat; add garlic and rosemary. Cook until toasted, 1–2 minutes.

2. Transfer toasted garlic and beans to a food processor with lemon juice and 2 tablespoons water. Purée until smooth; drizzle with additional oil before serving, if desired, and garnish with rosemary. Serve with pita chips.

Serving size: 3⅓ tablespoons dip and 1 ounce pita chips
Calories 225; Fat 7g (sat 0.4g, mono 1.7g, poly 0.3g); Cholesterol 0mg; Protein 7g; Carbohydrate 33g; Sugars 1g; Fiber 3g; RS 2g; Sodium 437mg

TIP:
This dip also works great as a Resistant Starch–packed sandwich spread. Make extra and refrigerate for up to 3 days.

RS
0.8g

Potato Canapés Stuffed with Sour Cream and Smoked Trout

Prep: *5 minutes* | **Cook:** *20 minutes* | **Total time:** *25 minutes* | **Makes:** *16 canapés*

Elegant enough for a fancy cocktail party, we love that these potatoes take less than 30 minutes to make. The trout filling is the perfect interplay of salty and creamy.

¾ pound mini red potatoes (about 8)

3 ounces pepper-crusted smoked trout, flaked

2 tablespoons light mayonnaise

1 tablespoon reduced calorie sour cream

1 tablespoon fresh lemon juice

2 tablespoons chopped chives, plus more for garnish

1. Place potatoes in a steamer and steam until tender but not mushy, 18–20 minutes. Cool, then halve.

2. Using the small side of a melon baller, carefully scoop out the centers of the potato halves and discard or reserve for another use.

3. Combine trout, mayonnaise, sour cream, lemon juice, and chives in a bowl.

4. Place potato halves on a large plate or platter. Scoop about 1½ teaspoons trout mixture into each hollowed-out potato half and sprinkle with some chopped chives.

Serving size: 4 canapés Calories 136; Fat 5.7g (sat 1.5g, mono 0.7g, poly 1.4g); Cholesterol 29mg; Protein 8g; Carbohydrate 14g; Sugars 1g; Fiber 1g; RS 0.8g; Sodium 396mg

TIP:
Look for smoked trout in the deli section of your grocery store. It's usually right by the smoked salmon.

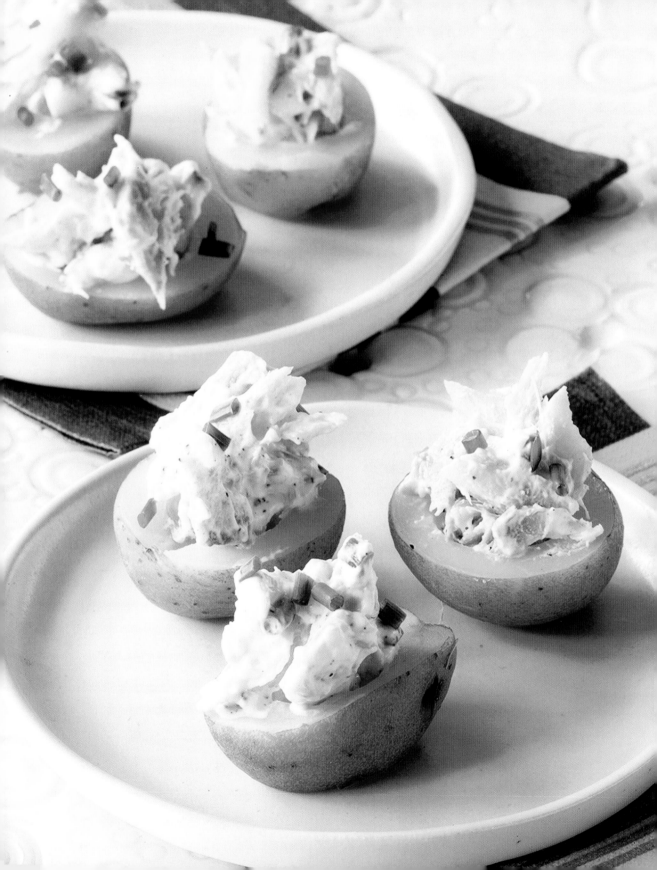

Mulled Cranberry Cocktail

Mint Mojito

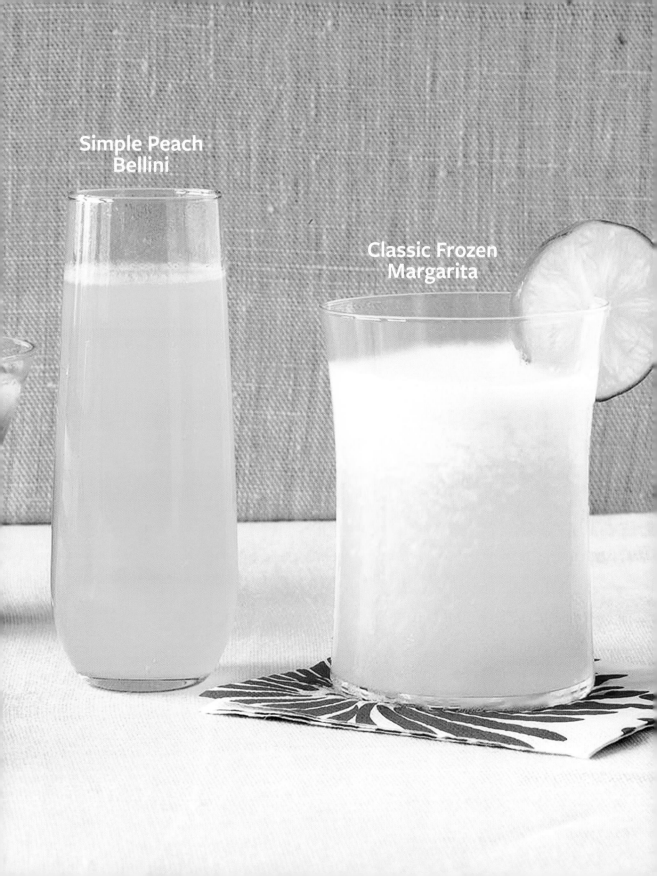

Simple Peach
Bellini

Classic Frozen
Margarita

Celebration Cocktails

Once you're on the 21-Day Immersion Plan, you can enjoy one of these cocktails.

Mulled Cranberry Cocktail

Prep: *5 minutes* **Cook:** *5 minutes*
Total Time: *40 minutes*
Makes: *5 servings*

- 4 cups cranberry juice, chilled, divided
- ½ cup brown sugar
- 2 strips orange zest
- 2 cinnamon sticks
- 4 cloves
- ½ teaspoon pure vanilla extract
- ¾ cup rum
- ¼ teaspoon orange bitters, optional

1. Combine 2 cups cranberry juice, sugar, zest, cinnamon, and cloves in a saucepan.

2. Simmer over medium heat until sugar dissolves. Let stand about 30 minutes.

3. Strain into a pitcher; stir in vanilla, rum, bitters (if using), and remaining 2 cups cranberry juice. Divide among 5 ice-filled glasses.

Serving size: 1 cup Calories 234; Fat 0g (sat 0g, mono 0g, poly 0g); Cholesterol 0mg; Protein 1g; Carbohydrate 37g; Sugars 29g; Fiber 0g; RS 0g; Sodium 11mg

Classic Frozen Margarita

Prep: *10 minutes*
Total Time: *2 hours 10 minutes*
Makes: *5 servings*

- ¼ cup triple sec
- ¾ cup lime juice
- ¼ cup water
- ½ cup orange juice
- ½ cup agave nectar
- ⅔ cup tequila

1. Combine triple sec, lime juice, water, orange juice, and agave in a pitcher.

2. Pour into an ice cube tray; freeze until just firm. Transfer ice cubes and tequila to a blender; blend until smooth. Divide among 5 glasses.

Serving size: about 1 cup Calories 219; Fat 0.1g (sat 0g, mono 0g, poly 0g); Cholesterol 0mg; Protein 0g; Carbohydrate 36g; Sugars 33g; Fiber 0g; RS 0g; Sodium 2mg

Mint Mojito

Prep: *5 minutes*
Total Time: *5 minutes*
Makes: *4 servings*

- 1 cup fresh mint leaves, plus more for garnish
- ⅓ cup agave nectar
- ¾ cup white rum
- 1 cup ice cubes
- 1 cup fresh lime juice
- 1 cup sparkling water

1. Combine mint, agave, rum, and ice cubes in pitcher.

2. Mash mint leaves, rum and agave together; stir in lime juice and water. Serve.

Serving size: 1 cup Calories 201; Fat 0.2g (sat 0.1g, mono 0g, poly 0.1g); Cholesterol 0mg; Protein 1g; Carbohydrate 28g; Sugars 22g; Fiber 2g; RS 0g; Sodium 8mg

Simple Peach Bellini

Prep: *3 minutes*
Total Time: *3 minutes*
Makes: *6 servings*

- 1½ cups peach nectar (such as Looza brand), chilled
- 1 (750-milliliter) bottle Cava or other sparkling wine, chilled

1. Divide peach nectar among 6 glasses; top with Cava.

2. Serve immediately.

Serving size: About 3/4 cup Calories 140; Fat 0g (sat 0g, mono 0g, poly 0g); Cholesterol 0mg; Protein 0g; Carbohydrate 12g; Sugars 10g; Fiber 1g; RS 0g; Sodium 3mg

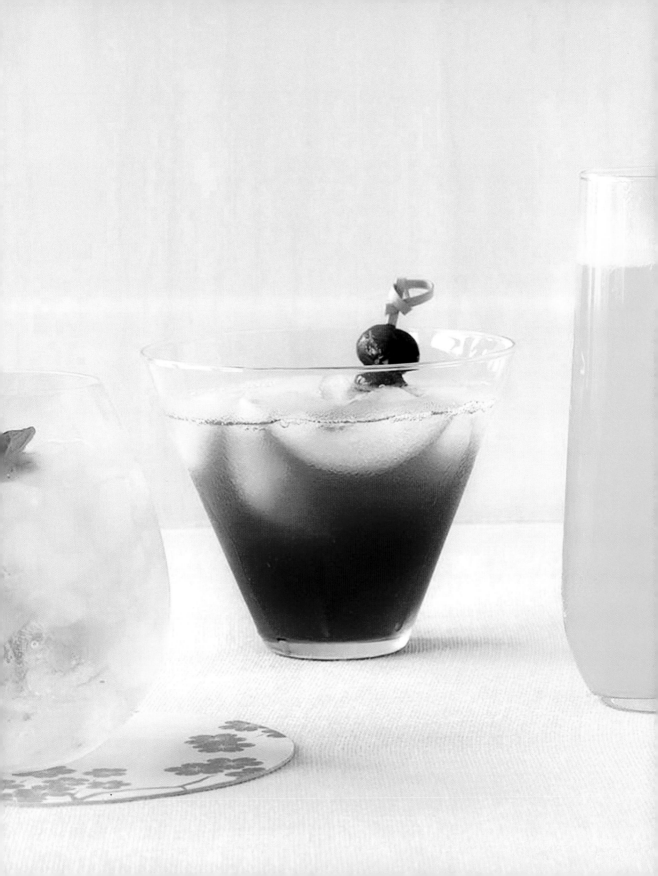

Dessert

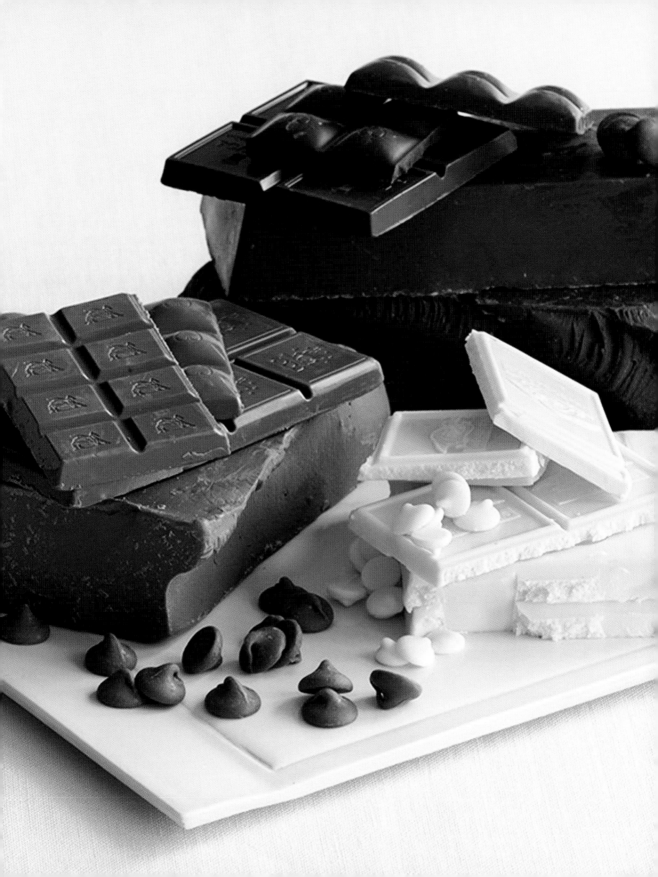

Rich Chocolate Pudding

Prep: *5 minutes* | **Cook:** *15 minutes* | **Total time:** *20 minutes + cooling time* | **Makes:** *4 servings*

Chocolate pudding is the ultimate comfort food indulgence. Ours uses bittersweet chocolate and unsweetened cocoa powder for a more intense chocolatey flavor.

2   ounces semisweet chocolate bar, divided
⅔   cup granulated sugar
¼   cup cornstarch
2   tablespoons unsweetened cocoa powder
¼   teaspoon salt
2½ cups skim milk
1   teaspoon pure vanilla extract
1   tablespoon butter

1. Using a vegetable peeler, shave 1 tablespoon curls from edge of chocolate bar (about ½ ounce). Chop remaining chocolate.

2. Combine sugar, cornstarch, cocoa, and salt in a medium saucepan. Gradually whisk in milk; bring to a boil over medium heat, whisking constantly, then boil, whisking, 2 minutes. Remove from heat; whisk in vanilla, butter, and chopped chocolate.

3. Divide pudding among 4 cups and cool for 30 minutes. Top with chocolate curls and serve.

Serving size: ¾ cup Calories 333; Fat 8.4g (sat 5.3g, mono 0.8g, poly 0.1g); Cholesterol 11mg; Protein 7g; Carbohydrate 58g; Sugars 47g; Fiber 1g; RS 0g; Sodium 211mg

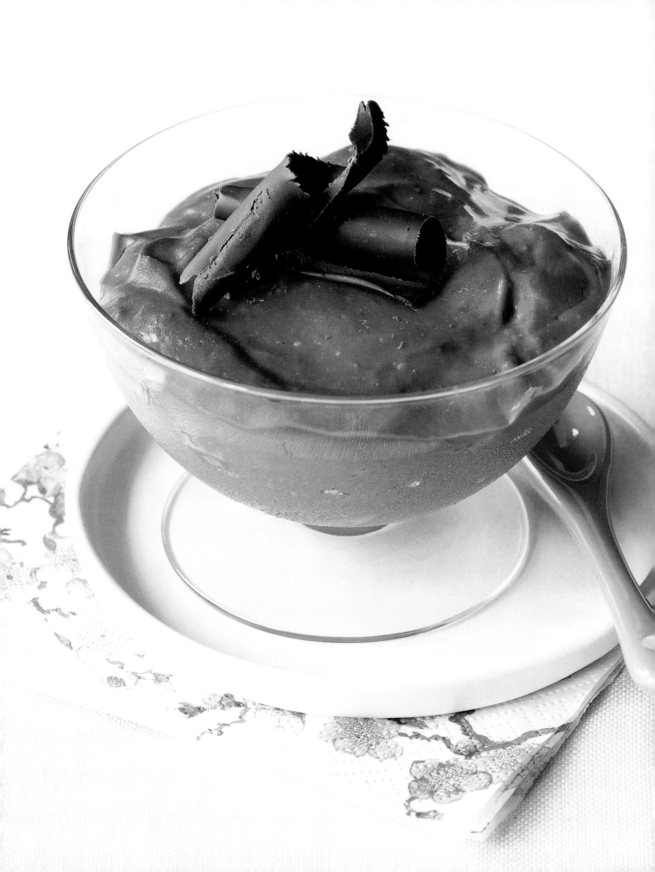

RS
2g

Old-Fashioned Banana Pudding

Prep: *10 minutes* | ***Cook/Assembly:*** *55 minutes* | ***Total time:*** *1 hour 5 minutes* | ***Makes:*** *8 servings*

This traditional Southern dessert is rich, creamy, and downright decadent. We lightened up the custard and used a yogurt cream instead of the usual whipped cream, but it's still just as homey and delicious.

¼ cup heavy whipping cream
½ cup fat-free Greek yogurt
½ cup sugar, divided
3 cups cold low-fat (1%) milk
5 tablespoons cornstarch
3 eggs
1 tablespoon pure vanilla extract
3 large bananas, sliced
  (about 2½ cups)
9 crumbled ladyfingers, divided

1. Whip cream until soft peaks are formed, 2 minutes. Fold in yogurt and 1 tablespoon of the sugar and refrigerate until ready to use (you will have about 1⅓ cups cream mixture). Whisk together milk, remaining sugar, cornstarch, eggs, and vanilla and pour into a saucepan. Bring to a boil, whisking often, then reduce the heat to a simmer and cook, whisking often, until custard has thickened, 9–10 minutes. Pour the custard into an 8- by 10-inch glass dish, cover surface with plastic wrap, and chill until cool, 40–45 minutes.

2. Reserve 8 banana slices and 1 crumbled ladyfinger for garnish. Place about ¼ cup of the custard on the bottom of a small drinking glass or parfait glass. Layer 2 tablespoons of the bananas, 1½ tablespoons of the yogurt-cream mixture, then 1 crumbled ladyfinger. Top with 2 tablespoons sliced bananas, ¼ cup custard, and 1 tablespoon yogurt-cream mixture. Top with a few ladyfinger crumbles and a banana slice.

Serving size: 1 pudding parfait Calories 249; Fat 5.9g (sat 3g, mono 1.8g, poly 0.5g); Cholesterol 92mg; Protein 8g; Carbohydrate 42g; Sugars 27g; Fiber 2g; RS 2g; Sodium 92mg

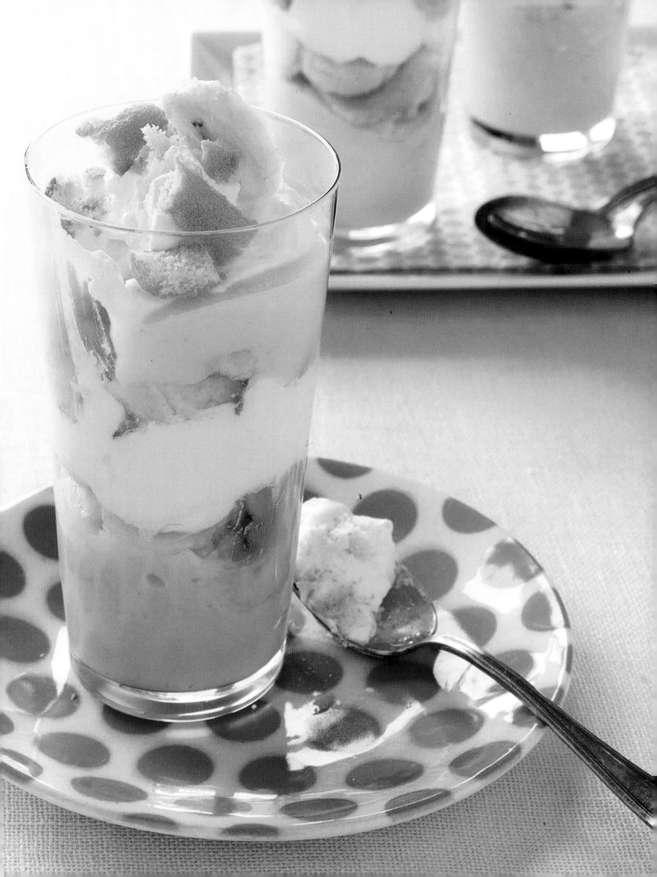

RS
1.2g

Banana-Walnut Loaf with Sour Cream Glaze

Prep: 15 minutes | Cook: 55 minutes | Total: 1 hour 5 minutes | Makes: 14 slices

Supermoist and packed full of toasty walnuts, this is no run-of-the-mill banana bread. Enjoy it with your afternoon tea or coffee.

Cooking spray
¾ cup all-purpose flour
¾ cup whole wheat flour
⅓ cup granulated sugar
1 teaspoon baking soda
½ teaspoon baking powder
1 teaspoon cinnamon
½ teaspoon ground nutmeg
¼ teaspoon salt
3 large, very ripe bananas, peeled and mashed (about 1½ cups)
⅓ cup vegetable oil
⅓ cup plus 1 tablespoon light sour cream, divided
¼ cup unsweetened applesauce
1 large egg
1 large egg white
1 teaspoon pure vanilla extract
⅓ cup toasted chopped walnuts
¼ cup powdered sugar

1. Preheat oven to 350°. Coat a 9- x 5-inch loaf pan with cooking spray and set aside.

2. Whisk together flours, sugar, baking soda, baking powder, cinnamon, nutmeg, and salt in a medium bowl. Whisk together bananas, oil, ⅓ cup sour cream, applesauce, eggs, and vanilla in a separate bowl.

3. Add wet ingredients to dry ingredients and mix until combined, then stir in walnuts until incorporated. Pour into prepared pan and bake for 55–60 minutes, or until a wooden skewer comes out clean. Cool completely.

4. Combine powdered sugar and remaining 1 tablespoon sour cream and whisk until smooth. Drizzle over banana bread and cut into 14 equal slices.

Serving size: 1 slice banana bread Calories 186; Fat 8.7g (sat 1.3g, mono 2g, poly 4.9g); Cholesterol 16mg; Protein 3.3g; Carbohydrate 25g; Sugars 11g; Fiber 2g; RS 1.2g; Sodium 166mg

ASK CARBLOVERS

Q: **I love sweets! How can I indulge in dessert without going overboard?**

A: Here are some tricks to help you practice moderation. First, make sure to put away any extra cookies, pudding, cake, etc. that haven't been eaten. And put freezable items in the back of the freezer (and out of sight!).

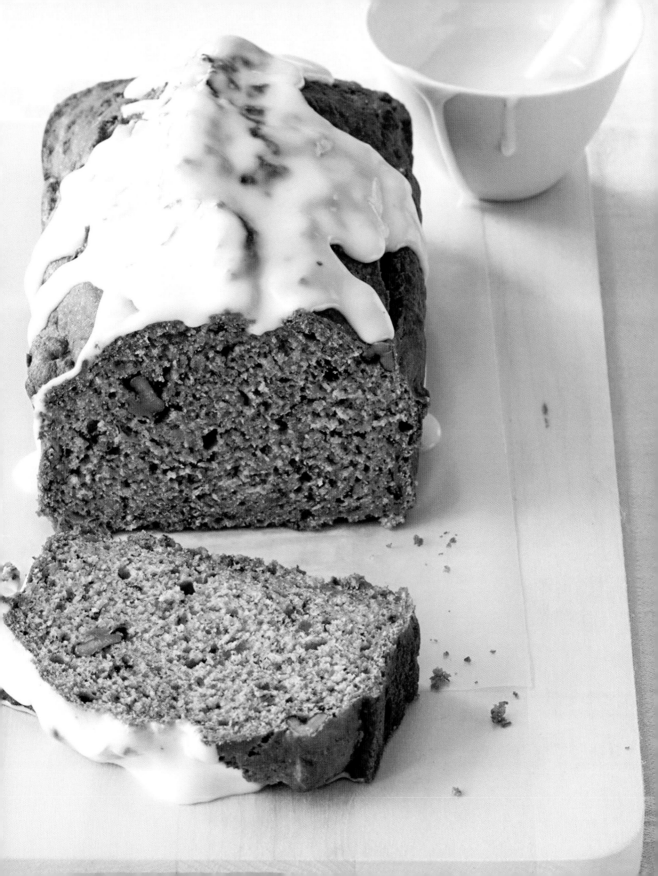

RS
0.9g

White Chocolate Banana Cream Pie

Prep: *15 minutes* | **Cook:** *20 minutes* | **Total time:** *35 minutes + 30 minutes cooling* | **Makes:** *10 servings*

We made this luscious dessert even more divine by adding a layer of white chocolate on top of the crust. Make it for your next dinner party or potluck—it's a showstopper!

1 (9-inch) store-bought graham-cracker pie shell
2 ounces white chocolate, melted and cooled
2 bananas, sliced (10 ounces)
½ cup granulated sugar
¼ cup light brown sugar
⅓ cup plus 2 teaspoons cornstarch, divided
¼ teaspoon salt
3 cups reduced-fat (2%) milk
1 teaspoon pure vanilla extract
1 tablespoon butter
2 large egg whites, at room temperature
¾ cup powdered sugar

1. Brush bottom and sides of pie shell with white chocolate. Place bananas in shell and transfer to refrigerator.

2. Combine sugars, ⅓ cup cornstarch, and salt in a medium saucepan. Gradually whisk in milk; bring to a boil over medium heat, whisking constantly, then boil, whisking, 2 minutes. Whisk in vanilla and butter. Transfer pudding to a bowl. Cover with plastic, directly touching surface of pudding, and cool until just warm, about 30 minutes. Pour cooled pudding into shell.

3. Preheat broiler, with rack in middle position. Beat egg whites and remaining 2 teaspoons cornstarch in the bowl of an electric mixer until soft peaks form. Gradually add powdered sugar until stiff peaks form, about 5–8 minutes. Spoon meringue over pudding to meet edge of pie shell and swirl with a spoon. Broil pie until browned in spots, rotating pie occasionally, about 2–3 minutes.

Serving size: 1 slice pie Calories 288; Fat 7.3g (sat 3.2g, mono 1.2g, poly 0.2g); Cholesterol 10mg; Protein 5g; Carbohydrate 53g; Sugars 39g; Fiber 1g; RS 0.9g; Sodium 191mg

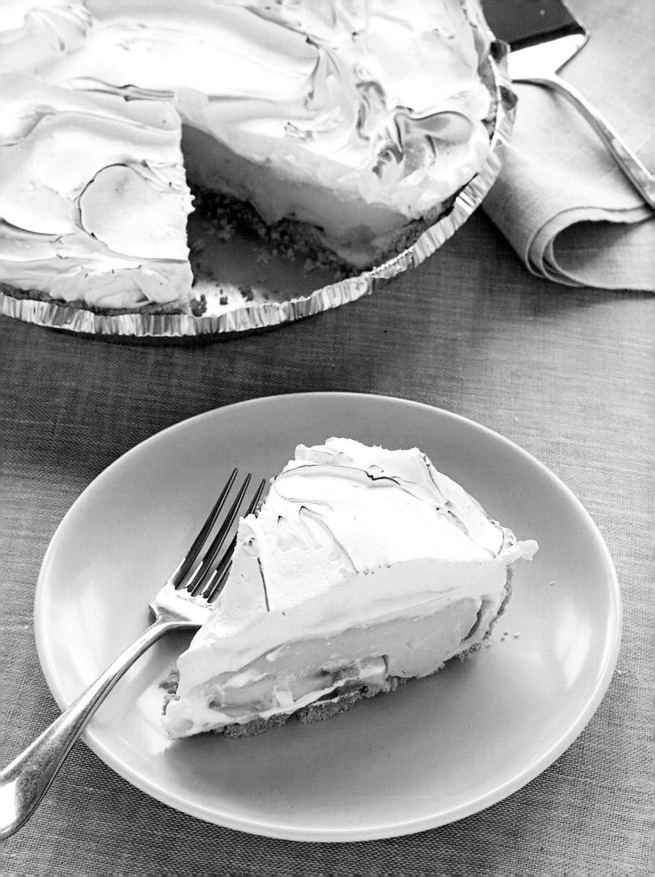

Bananas Foster

RS
4.7g

Prep: *5 minutes* | **Cook:** *10 minutes* | **Total time:** *15 minutes* | **Makes:** *4 servings*

Created in New Orleans in the 1950s, this easy—yet impressive—dessert is legendary. Not only is it delicious, a single serving also has nearly 5 grams of Resistant Starch.

3 tablespoons butter
⅓ cup light brown sugar
½ teaspoon pure vanilla extract
¼ teaspoon cinnamon
⅛ teaspoon salt
4 ripe bananas, halved lengthwise
¼ cup dark rum
2 cups low-fat vanilla frozen yogurt (optional)

1. Melt butter in a large skillet over medium-low heat. Add brown sugar, vanilla, cinnamon, and salt; cook, stirring, until brown sugar melts, 2–3 minutes.

2. Raise heat to medium, add bananas, and cook, stirring, until caramelized on all sides, 3–4 minutes. Remove pan from flame, add rum and very carefully light with a match to ignite the alcohol. Shake carefully until flame dies (if you like a thicker sauce you can return the pan to the stove for an additional 1–2 minutes).

2. Divide bananas among 4 bowls and top with ½ cup frozen yogurt, if desired. Serve immediately.

Serving size: 1 banana, 2 tablespoons butter-rum sauce
Calories 285; Fat 9g (sat 5.6g, mono 2.3g, poly 0.4g); Cholesterol 23mg; Protein 1g; Carbohydrate 45g; Sugars 32g; Fiber 3g; RS 4.7g; Sodium 80mg

TIP:
Caramelized bananas make an amazing topping for waffles and French toast. Just slice the bananas instead of halving lengthwise.

Holiday Chocolate Bark

Prep: *5 minutes* | ***Cook:*** *10 minutes* | ***Total time:*** *15 minutes + 30 minutes chilling* | ***Makes:*** *15 servings*

Great to give as a gift to friends and family during the holidays, this chocolate bark is bursting with the season's richest flavors.

6   ounces semisweet chocolate
6   ounces bittersweet chocolate
¼   teaspoon salt
⅛   teaspoon ground cinnamon
½   cup puffed brown-rice cereal
⅔   cup chopped pistachios
     (3 ounces), divided
⅔   cup chopped dried cherries,
     divided
2   ounces white chocolate, melted

1. Line a rimmed 15- by 10-inch baking sheet with foil; refrigerate.

2. Melt chocolates with salt and cinnamon in a large heat-safe bowl set over simmering water, stirring often. Stir in cereal and half of pistachios and cherries. Immediately pour onto prepared baking sheet and spread with a spatula into a large rectangle, about ¼-inch thick. Sprinkle with remaining pistachios and cherries; drizzle with white chocolate.

2. Refrigerate until firm, about 30 minutes. To serve, break into pieces. To store, transfer to an airtight container and refrigerate up to 3 days.

Serving size: About 1 ounce Calories 198; Fat 12.7g (sat 6.2g, mono 1.7g, poly 0.8g); Cholesterol 1mg; Protein 3g; Carbohydrate 21g; Sugars 14g; Fiber 2g; RS 0g; Sodium 47mg

Mini Chocolate-Cinnamon Molten Cakes

Prep: 15 minutes | **Cook:** 12 minutes | **Total time:** 27 minutes | **Makes:** 8 servings

Warm and rich, this little pot of goodness is a chocolate lover's dream. If you've never made molten cakes before, go ahead and give them a try—they're easier than you think!

Cooking spray
¾ cup whole wheat pastry flour
½ cup unsweetened natural cocoa powder
1½ teaspoons baking powder
⅛ teaspoon salt
5 tablespoons butter, room temperature
½ cup sugar
2 eggs and 2 egg whites (¾ cup liquid)
2 teaspoons pure vanilla extract
2 ounces high-quality dark chocolate, melted
1 tablespoon espresso powder, dissolved in 1 teaspoon hot water
2 tablespoons powdered sugar
Mixed berries and whipped cream, for serving (optional)

1. Preheat oven to 350°. Coat eight 4-ounce ramekins with cooking spray and place on a baking sheet; set aside.

2. Sift flour, cocoa, baking powder, and salt into a bowl.

3. In the bowl of an electric mixer, using the paddle attachment, cream butter and sugar until light and fluffy. Add eggs, egg whites and vanilla and beat until incorporated, 1 minute. Add flour mixture to butter-sugar mixture, and gently mix to combine. Add melted chocolate and dissolved espresso and gently fold in. Divide the batter into the prepared ramekins.

4. Bake until cakes are puffy and cracked on top but still gooey in the middle, 12–13 minutes. Remove from oven and sift powdered sugar over the top. Serve warm, with berries or cream, if desired.

Serving size: 1 cake Calories 232; Fat 11.4g (sat 6.6g, mono 2.3g, poly 0.5g); Cholesterol 66mg; Protein 5g; Carbohydrate 29g; Sugars 17g; Fiber 2g; RS 0g; Sodium 172mg

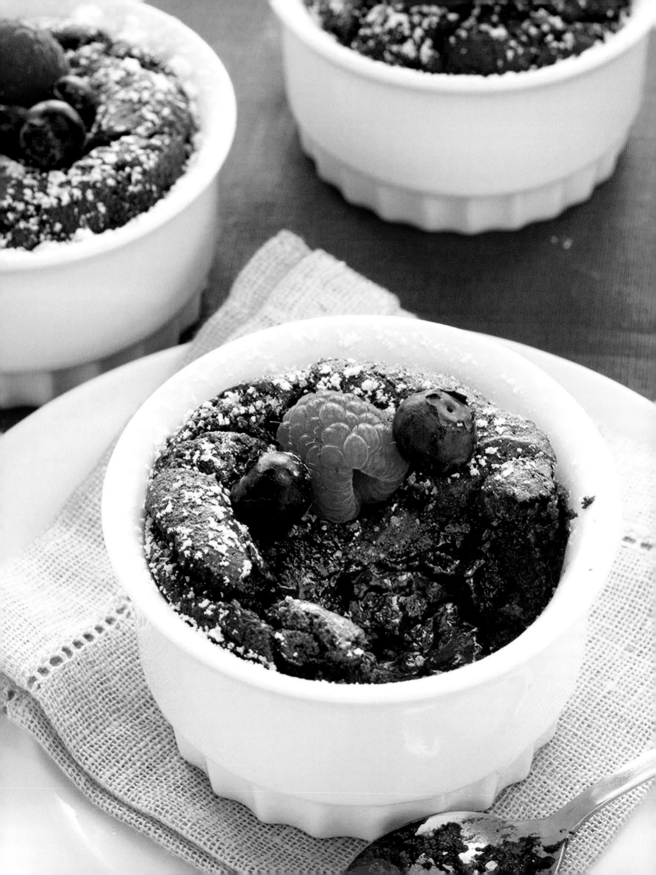

Coconut Cake with 7-Minute Frosting

Prep: *20 minutes* | **Cook:** *30–33 minutes + time for frosting* |
Total time: *55 minutes + 1 hour cooling* | **Makes:** *14 servings*

This gorgeous celebration cake deserves to be center stage at your next gathering.
We used tofu to help lower the fat, but we won't tell if you don't!

Cooking spray
1 cup plus ½ cup sugar, divided
½ cup shredded unsweetened
coconut, plus more for serving
2½ cups all-purpose flour, spooned
and leveled, plus more for dusting
2½ teaspoons baking powder
½ teaspoon table salt
3 ounces extra-firm tofu (⅓ cup)
¾ cup light coconut milk
1 teaspoon pure vanilla extract
½ cup vegetable oil

FOR FROSTING:

3 large egg whites
1½ cups sugar
¼ teaspoon cream of tartar
Dash of salt
1 teaspoon vanilla extract

1. Preheat oven to 350°. Coat two 8-inch round baking pans with cooking spray and line with parchment. Coat with spray; dust with flour.

2. Combine ½ cup sugar, ½ cup water, and coconut in a saucepan. Simmer until sugar dissolves, 2–3 minutes; cover and set aside. Strain and reserve coconut and syrup separately.

3. Combine flour, baking powder, and salt in a large bowl. In a blender, combine tofu, coconut milk, vanilla, oil, reserved coconut and remaining 1 cup sugar; blend until smooth. Add wet ingredients to dry ingredients and stir. Divide batter between baking pans and spread evenly; bake until edges begin to pull away from sides of pan, 25–30 minutes.

4. Cool 5 minutes in pans; invert onto a wire rack to cool completely. As cake cools, brush with reserved coconut syrup.

5. Make frosting: Place first 4 ingredients (through salt) in a large deep heatproof bowl set over about 1½ inches of simmering water; beat with a handheld electric mixer at low speed. Increase to medium-high, beating until peaks form when beaters are lifted (about 7 minutes). Remove bowl from saucepan; continue beating until frosting is cool (about 3 minutes). Beat in vanilla. Frost cakes; sprinkle with coconut.

Serving size: 1 slice cake Calories 370; Fat 12.1g (sat 3.8g, mono 2g, poly 5.4g); Cholesterol 0mg; Protein 4g; Carbohydrate 62g; Sugars 44g; Fiber 1g; RS 0g; Sodium 202mg

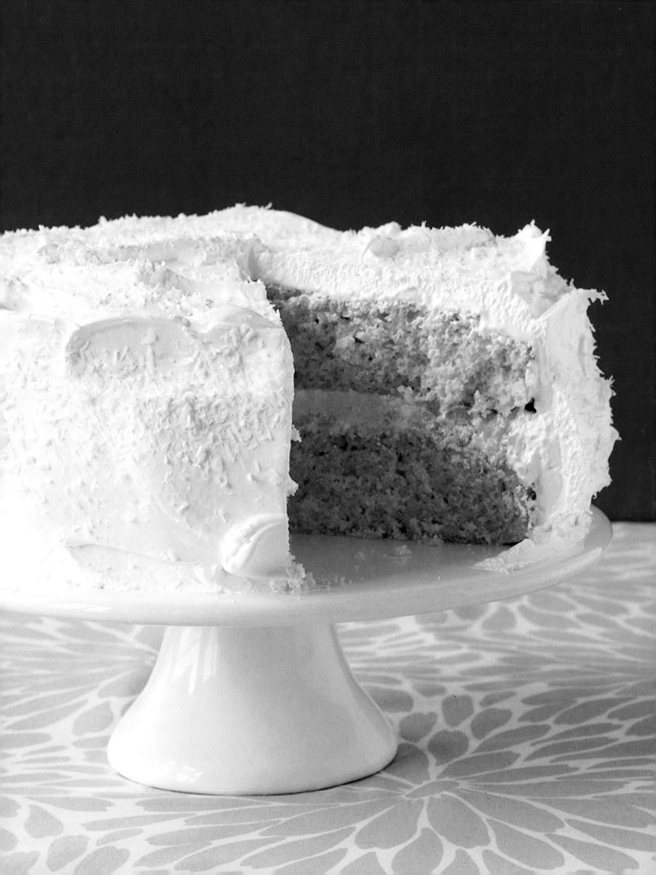

RS
1.1g

Oatmeal-Date-Chocolate Cookies

Prep: *10 minutes* | **Cook:** *12 minutes* | **Total time:** *22 minutes* | **Makes:** *32 cookies*

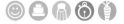

Chocolate chip cookies are the ultimate feel-good treat. And you'll feel even better about these because they're made with high-fiber dates and oats and chocolate chunks.

6	tablespoons unsalted butter
¾	cup packed light brown sugar
⅓	cup all-purpose flour
⅓	cup whole wheat flour
¾	teaspoon baking soda
1½	cups regular oats
½	teaspoon salt
1	egg, lightly beaten
1	teaspoon pure vanilla extract
1	cup chopped pitted dates
3	ounces coarsely chopped bittersweet chocolate

1. Preheat oven to 350º.

2. Melt butter in a small saucepan over low heat. Remove from heat and stir in brown sugar until smooth. Combine flours, baking soda, oats, and salt in a medium bowl. Combine the butter mixture with the dry ingredients, and add egg, vanilla, and dates. Fold in chocolate.

3. Mix well and spoon mixture by tablespoonfuls onto lightly greased (or parchment paper–lined) baking sheets. Bake for 12 minutes, until tops are dry to the touch. Cool completely on wire rack.

Serving size: 1 cookie Calories 93; Fat 3.8g (sat 2.2g, mono 0.7g, poly 0.2g); Cholesterol 12mg; Protein 1g;Carbohydrate 14g; Sugars 9g; Fiber 1g, RS 1.1g; Sodium 70mg

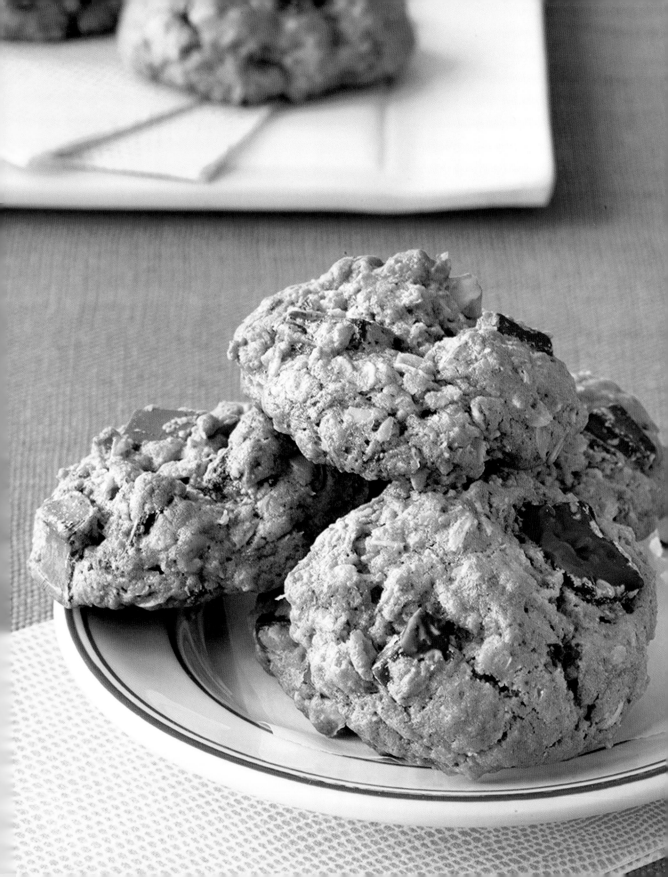

Toasted Almond-Caramel Popcorn Clusters

Rocky Road Rice Krispy Treats

**Pecan
Blondies**

**Chocolate
Brownie Bites**

RS
0–1.1g

CarbLovers Sweets

Have you ever seen a diet cookbook that featured so many delicous baked treats? Make a batch to share at your next book club meeting or girls' night in.

Toasted Almond-Caramel Popcorn Clusters

Prep: 5 minutes
Cook: 12 minutes
Total time: 17 minutes
Makes: 8 servings

Cooking spray
8 individually wrapped caramel candies, unwrapped
⅛ teaspoon salt
2 cups air-popped popcorn
2 tablespoons toasted unsalted chopped almonds

1. Coat foil-lined baking sheet with cooking spray; set aside.

2. Place caramels in double boiler and stir over medium heat until melted. Add salt and almonds and stir to combine. Add popcorn. Working quickly, stir to incorporate popcorn into caramel mixture.

3. Coat a ¼-cup measure with cooking spray. Scoop popcorn mixture ¼ cup at a time and drop onto prepared sheet; let cool until easy to handle, about 20 seconds. Roll into balls and let cool.

Serving size: 1 cluster Calories 58; Fat 2g (sat 0.3g, mono 0.7g, poly 0.6g); Cholesterol 1mg; Protein 1g; Carbohydrate 10g; Sugars 7g; Fiber 1g; RS 0g: Sodium 61mg

Rocky Road Rice Krispy Treats

Prep: 10 minutes
Cook: 10 minutes
Total time: 20 minutes + 30 minutes cooling
Makes: 15 bars

Cooking spray
1 (10½-ounce) bag miniature marshmallows, divided
4 tablespoons unsalted butter
¼ cup unsweetened cocoa powder
6 cups crispy brown rice cereal
½ cup chopped almonds
2 ounces semisweet chocolate, chopped and melted

1. Coat a 9- by 13-inch pan with cooking spray; set aside. Reserve 1 cup marshmallows.

2. Combine butter, cocoa, and remaining marshmallows in a large pot; cook over medium-low heat until marshmallows are melted, 3–5 minutes. Add rice cereal, almonds, and reserved marshmallows to mixture; stir until combined and sticky.

3. Press into prepared pan and drizzle with melted chocolate. Chill in refrigerator 30 minutes. Cut into 15 (2½ - by 3-inch) bars; serve.

Serving size: 1 rectangle Calories 176; Fat 6.8g (sat 3g, mono 2g, poly 0.6g); Cholesterol 8mg; Protein 2g; Carbohydrate 27g; Sugars 14g; Fiber 1g; RS 0.2g; Sodium 67mg

Chocolate Brownie Bites

Prep: 10 minutes
Cook: 10 minutes
Total time: 20 minutes
Makes: 12 servings

Cooking spray
3 ounces semisweet chocolate, finely chopped
3 tablespoons butter
2 teaspoons espresso powder, dissolved in 1 tablespoon warm water
1 teaspoon pure vanilla extract
¼ cup all-purpose flour
1 large egg, lightly beaten
3 tablespoons sugar
3 tablespoons light brown sugar

1. Preheat oven to 350°. Coat a mini muffin pan with cooking spray and set aside. Melt chocolate and butter in a small saucepan over low heat, stirring until smooth. Remove from heat, transfer to a medium bowl and add dissolved espresso and vanilla.

2. Add flour to chocolate mixture and stir well. Add egg and stir to incorporate. Add sugars and stir until smooth. Spoon batter evenly into prepared pan. Bake until just cooked through and tops are smooth and slightly puffy, 10–12 minutes.

3. Cool completely (as bites cool, they will collapse and tops will invert) and enjoy.

Serving size: 1 brownie bite Calories 111; Fat 6.1g (sat 3.7g, mono 1.1g, poly 0.2g); Cholesterol 23mg; Protein 1g; Carbohydrate 13g; Sugars 9g; Fiber 0g; RS 0g; Sodium 8mg

Pecan Blondies

Prep: 10 minutes
Cook: 30 minutes
Total time: 40 minutes + cooling
Makes: 16 squares

Cooking spray
- ½ cup all-purpose flour, spooned and leveled
- ¾ cup old-fashioned rolled oats
- ⅔ cup packed light brown sugar
- ½ teaspoon salt
- 4 tablespoons butter, melted
- 2 tablespoons vegetable oil
- ¼ cup apple juice
- 1 large egg
- 2 teaspoons pure vanilla extract
- ¼ cup pecans, roughly chopped

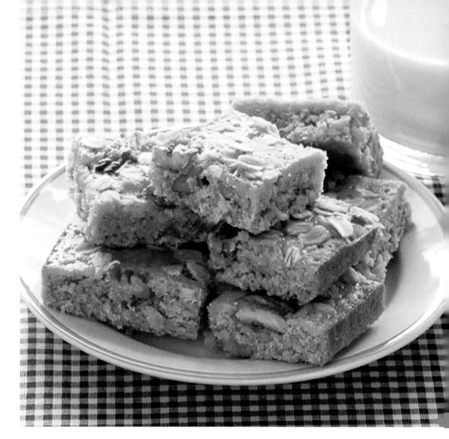

1. Preheat oven to 350°. Coat an 8-inch square baking pan with cooking spray; line with parchment (to overhang on two sides) and lightly coat parchment.

2. Combine flour, ½ cup oats, sugar, and salt in the bowl of a food processor; pulse until oats are finely ground. Add butter, oil, juice, egg, and vanilla; pulse until combined.

2. Transfer batter to prepared pan; sprinkle with pecans and remaining ¼ cup oats. Bake until edges pull away from sides of pan, 25 to 30 minutes. Transfer to a wire rack to cool completely; cut into 16 (2- by 2-inch) squares.

Serving size: One 2-inch square Calories 124; Fat 6.5g (sat 2.2g, mono 2.1g, poly 1.8g); Cholesterol 19mg; Protein 1g; Carbohydrate 15g; Sugars 10g; Fiber 1g; RS 1.1g; Sodium 81mg

Pavlova with Fresh Strawberries

Prep: *20 minutes* | **Cook:** *1 hour 30 minutes* | **Total time:** *1 hour 50 minutes + standing time* |
Makes: *4 servings*

This popular meringue dessert was created in the 1920s for the Russian ballet dancer Anna Pavlova, and is just as light and airy as a grand jeté.

¾ cup powdered sugar
1 tablespoon cornstarch
4 egg whites, at room temperature
¼ teaspoon cream of tartar
   Pinch of salt
¼ teaspoon pure vanilla extract
¼   cup heavy cream
2 tablespoons agave nectar, divided
1   tablespoon fresh lemon juice, plus ½ teaspoon finely grated zest
2 cups strawberries, hulled and halved

1. Preheat oven to 225°. Whisk together sugar and cornstarch; set aside. Beat egg whites at medium-high speed with a stand mixer for 1 minute; add cream of tartar and salt, beating until blended. Gradually add sugar mixture 1 tablespoon at a time, beating at medium-high speed until mixture is glossy, stiff peaks form, and sugar dissolves. (Do not overbeat.) Beat in vanilla. Gently spread mixture into a 7-inch round on a parchment-lined baking sheet, making an indentation in center of meringue to hold filling.

2. Bake for 1 hour and 30 minutes or until pale golden and the outside has formed a crust. Turn oven off; let meringue stand in oven, with door closed, 12 hours.

3. Before serving, whip cream until stiff peaks form; whisk in 1 tablespoon agave. In a separate bowl, whisk together remaining agave and lemon juice; toss with zest and berries.

4. Spoon whipped cream on top of meringue, and top with berries. (Center of meringue may fall once the lemon mixture and berries have been added.)

Serving size: ¼ of meringue, ½ cup berries, 2 tablespoons whipped cream Calories 219; Fat 5.8g (sat 3.5g, mono 1.6g, poly 0.3g); Cholesterol 21mg; Protein 4g; Carbohydrate 39g; Sugars 34g; Fiber 2g; RS 0g; Sodium 97mg

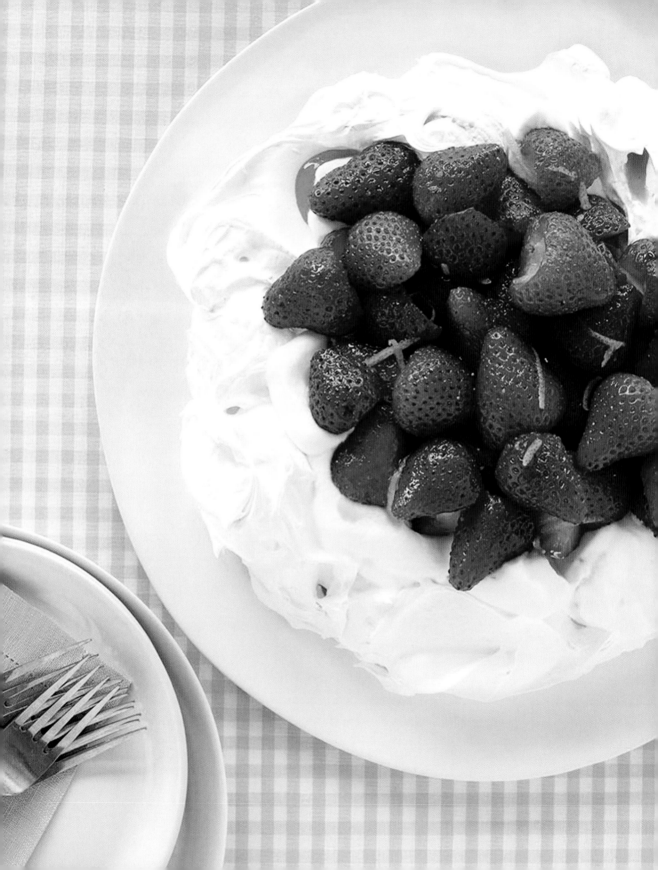

Bourbon Apple Crumble with Oats and Pecans

Prep: *15 minutes* | **Cook:** *45 minutes* | **Total time:** *1 hour* | **Makes:** *6 servings*

Sweet and fragrant with the luscious scent of spiced apples, this no-fail crumble makes a welcoming fall or winter dessert.

Cooking spray
4 medium Fuji apples (about 2 pounds), peeled and cut into 1-inch pieces
1 tablespoon bourbon
1 tablespoon plus ¼ cup all-purpose flour, divided
¼ cup regular oats, uncooked
¼ cup packed light brown sugar
½ teaspoon pumpkin pie spice
⅛ teaspoon salt
3 tablespoons chilled butter
¼ cup chopped pecans

1. Preheat oven to 375°.

2. Coat an 8-inch square baking dish with cooking spray. Combine apples, bourbon, and 1 tablespoon flour; arrange in prepared dish, pressing down lightly to compact.

3. Combine remaining ¼ cup flour, oats, sugar, pie spice, and salt in a medium bowl; cut in butter using a pastry blender or 2 knives until mixture resembles coarse meal. Stir in pecans. Sprinkle mixture over apples.

4. Bake for 45 minutes or until bubbly and golden brown. Serve warm.

Serving size: ⅔ cup crumble Calories 245; Fat 10.2g (sat 4.1g, mono 3.9g, poly 1.5g); Cholesterol 15mg; Protein 2g; Carbohydrate 38g; Sugars 25g; Fiber 5g; RS 1g; Sodium 54mg

TIP:
Make this dessert special for company: Spoon low-fat vanilla yogurt into parfait glasses, alternating crumble layers with yogurt, ending with the crumble. Dig in!

RS
2.4g

Chocolate Drizzled Crepes with Fresh Banana Jam

Prep: *5 minutes* | **Cook:** *5 minutes* | **Total time:** *10 minutes* | **Makes:** *4 servings*

Say oui *to these delicious crepes! Not only can you make them in just 10 minutes, they're packed with more than 2 grams of Resistant Starch.*

2   bananas, peeled and coarsely chopped
1½ cups fat-free milk
2   tablespoons sugar
4   (12-inch) prepared crepes (such as LeSter brand)
2   ounces bittersweet chocolate, melted

1. Mash bananas, milk, and sugar with a potato masher in a medium skillet to combine. Cook over medium heat, stirring, until thick and almost smooth, about 5 minutes.

2. Fill each crepe with ¼ cup of the banana mixture; fold into a triangle. Drizzle with chocolate and serve.

Serving size: 1 crepe with ¼ cup banana mixture
Calories 277; Fat 9.1g (sat 5.8g, mono 2.6g, poly 0.3g); Cholesterol 27mg; Protein 7g; Carbohydrate 46g; Sugars 28g; Fiber 3g; RS 2.4g; Sodium 236mg

Watermelon-Lime

Pineapple-Mint

Grapefruit-Prosecco

Icy, Refreshing Granitas

Prep: *5 minutes* | **Total time:** *2 hours 30 minutes* | **Makes:** *6 servings*

We love granitas because they're so light, refreshing, and incredibly low-cal. Experiment with your own flavor combinations!

Grapefruit–Prosecco

- 2 cups grapefruit juice
- 1 cup Prosecco or sparkling white grape juice
- 3 tablespoons agave nectar

Serving size: 1 cup Calories 95; Fat 0.1g (sat 0g, mono 0g, poly 0g); Cholesterol 0mg; Protein 0g; Carbohydrate 16g; Sugars 15g; Fiber 0g; RS 0g; Sodium 1mg

Pineapple-Mint

- 3 cups pineapple juice
- 3 tablespoons finely chopped mint
- 2 tablespoons fresh lemon juice
- 2 tablespoons agave nectar

Serving size: 1 cup Calories 87; Fat 0g (sat 0g, mono 0g, poly 0g); Cholesterol 0mg; Protein 0g; Carbohydrate 21g; Sugars 17g; Fiber 0g; RS 0g; Sodium 6mg

Watermelon-Lime

- 8 cups (2 pounds) seedless watermelon, blended and strained through a fine-mesh sieve, solids discarded (about 2¾ cups juice)
- 5 tablespoons fresh lime juice
- 3 tablespoons agave nectar

Serving size: 1 cup Calories 68; Fat 0g (sat 0g, mono 0g, poly 0g); Cholesterol 0mg; Protein 1g; Carbohydrate 19g; Sugars 16g; Fiber 1g; RS 0g; Sodium 3mg

1. Clear a large area in the freezer and place a 10- by 17-inch rimmed baking sheet inside. Combine all ingredients in a pitcher and carefully pour onto baking sheet in freezer.

2. After 1 hour scrape a fork across the surface of the liquid (which will be partially frozen but still very slushy). Scrape surface every 30 minutes for the next 90 minutes until mixture has separated into icy crystals. Scoop into parfait glasses, martini glasses, or glass dessert bowls.

TIP:
Make-ahead granitas? Sure. Just keep the mixture in an airtight container in your freezer for up to 2 weeks (mix with fork occasionally to keep icy consistency).

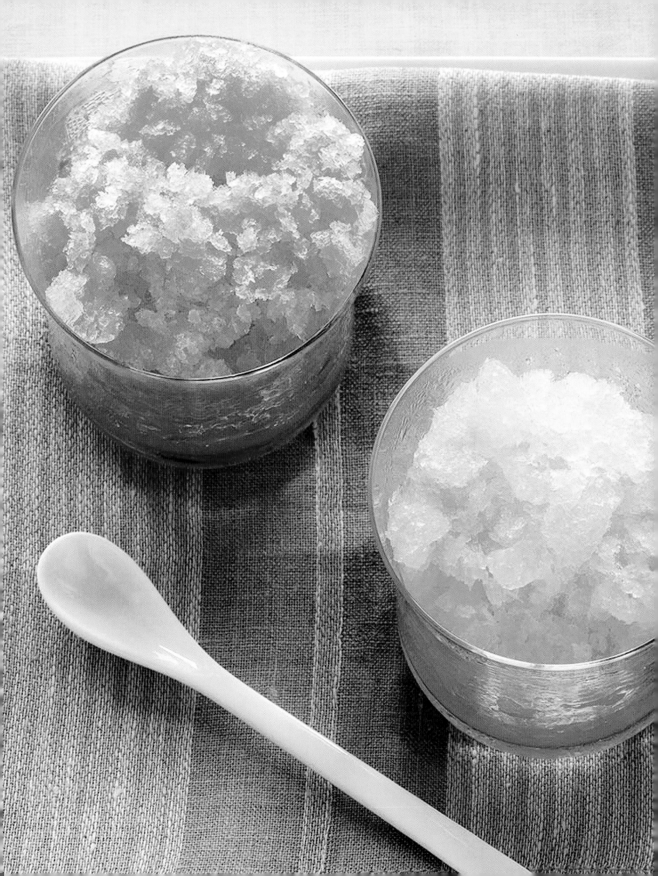

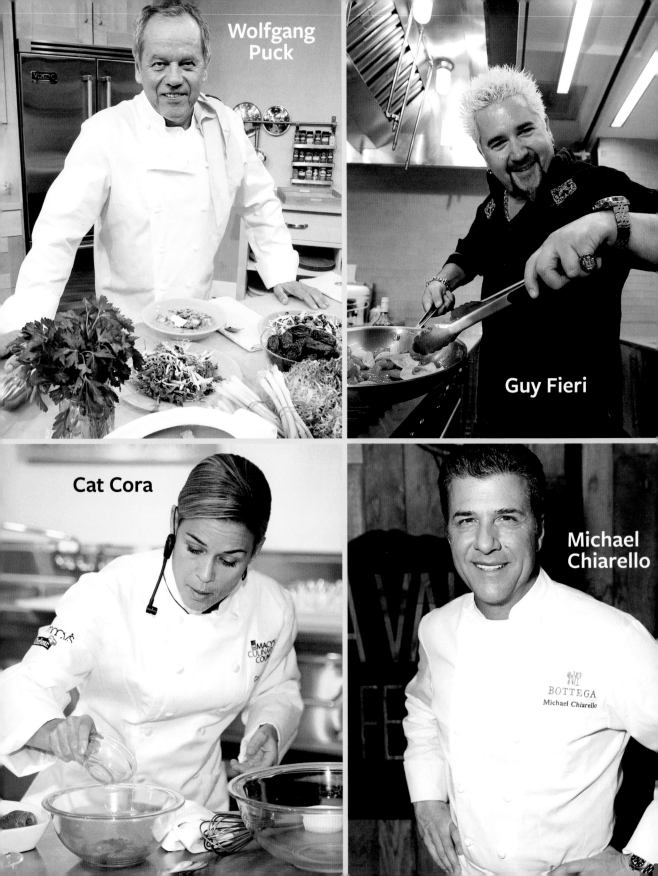

Wolfgang Puck

Guy Fieri

Cat Cora

Michael Chiarello

Star Chefs Cook Carbs!

RS
3.3g

Guy Fieri's Spinach-Tomato Pasta Shells

Prep: 5 minutes | **Cook:** 15 minutes | **Total time:** 20 minutes | **Makes:** 4 servings

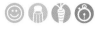

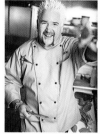

"I have to straight-up admit that I'm a pasta junkie. If you're gonna indulge in the greatest of carbs, at least fortify it with a little baby spinach. Not only is this dish healthy, but with the color from the tomatoes and spinach, it looks great as well."

Guy Fieri is the author of *Guy Fieri Food: Cookin' It, Livin' It, Lovin' It,* host of *Guy's Big Bite* and *Diners, Drive-ins and Dives* on Food Network, and founder of the nonprofit group, Cooking with Kids.

¾   pound whole wheat pasta shells
1   tablespoon butter
1   shallot, thinly sliced
¼   teaspoon crushed red pepper
1   (5-ounce) package baby spinach
½   cup low-sodium chicken broth
¼   cup half and half
1   ounce grated Pecorino Romano cheese, divided
½   teaspoon freshly ground black pepper
1   (8-ounce) container grape tomatoes, halved lengthwise
1   tablespoon chopped flat-leaf parsley

1. Cook pasta according to package directions.

2. Meanwhile, heat butter in a large skillet over medium-high heat. Add shallot and crushed red pepper; reduce heat to medium-low, and cook for 1–2 minutes or until translucent. Add spinach and broth; cover and cook for 1 minute. Add half-and-half, ¾ of the cheese, and the black pepper. Stir to combine; cook for 3 minutes. Remove from heat.

3. Add tomatoes and the cooked pasta; toss. Garnish with parsley and remaining cheese. Serve.

Serving size: about 2 cups Calories 402; Fat 7.8g (sat 4.4g, mono 2g, poly 0.7g); Cholesterol 21mg; Protein 17g; Carbohydrate 72g; Sugars 5g; Fiber 9g; Iron 4mg; RS 3.3g; Sodium 165mg

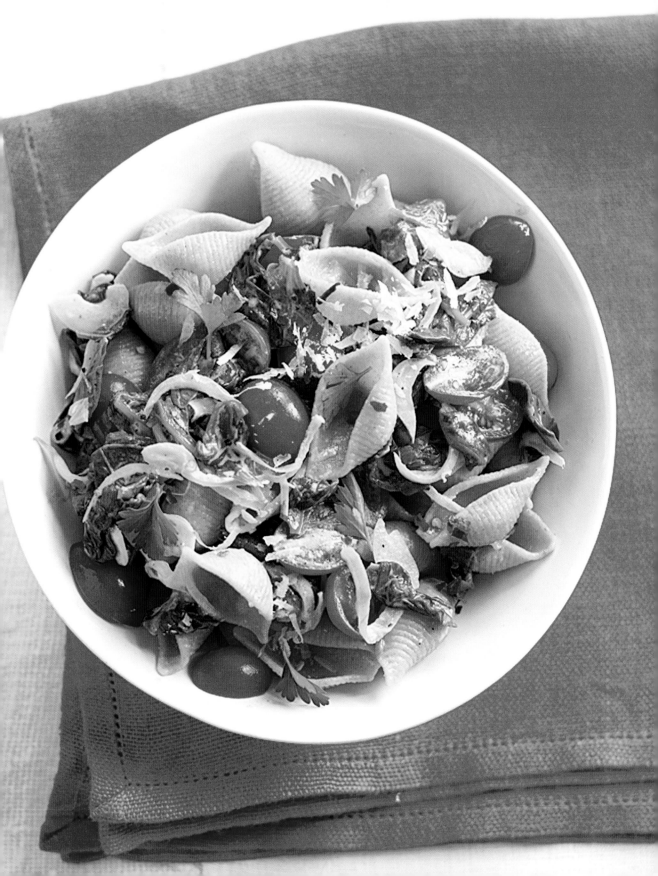

RS
2.6g

Wolfgang Puck's Barbecue Chicken Pizza

Prep: *10 minutes* | **Cook:** *15 minutes* | **Total time:** *25 minutes* | **Makes:** *5 servings*

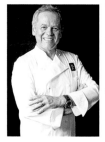

"I like this recipe because you can add grilled or sautéed vegetables to the toppings. Or try spinach, Swiss chard, or kale. Blanch in boiling salted water first, then drain, squeeze dry, chop, and top the pizza."

Wolfgang Puck is the master chef/owner of over 20 fine-dining establishments and more than 80 fast cafes and bistros around the world. In addition to his impressive restaurant portfolio, Puck has established catering operations in 16 major markets. He's also created a line of Wolfgang Puck housewares.

2 teaspoons olive oil
1 cup thinly sliced yellow and red
   bell peppers
   All-purpose flour for rolling
1 pound refrigerated pizza dough
½ cup grated mozzarella cheese
½ cup fontina cheese
1½ cups cooked chicken breast, cut
   into 1-inch pieces
¼ cup barbecue sauce, warmed
¼ teaspoon salt
¼ teaspoon pepper
¼ cup chopped flat-leaf parsley

1. Preheat oven to 500°.

2. Heat oil in a medium skillet over medium-high heat; sauté peppers for 2 minutes. Set aside. Roll out pizza dough to a 15-inch round on a lightly floured surface; top with cheeses and sautéed peppers. Transfer to a baking pan. Bake pizza for about 12 minutes or until crust is golden brown.

3. Meanwhile, warm up chicken. Toss warm chicken pieces with barbecue sauce. Remove pizza from the oven; evenly arrange chicken on top. Sprinkle with salt and pepper, and top with parsley. Cut pizza into slices; serve.

Serving size: ⅕ of pizza Calories 414; Fat 10.7g (sat 4g, mono 3.3g, poly 0.8g); Cholesterol 54mg; Protein 27g; Carbohydrate 49g; Sugars 6g; Fiber 7g; Iron 2mg; RS 2.6g; Sodium 804mg

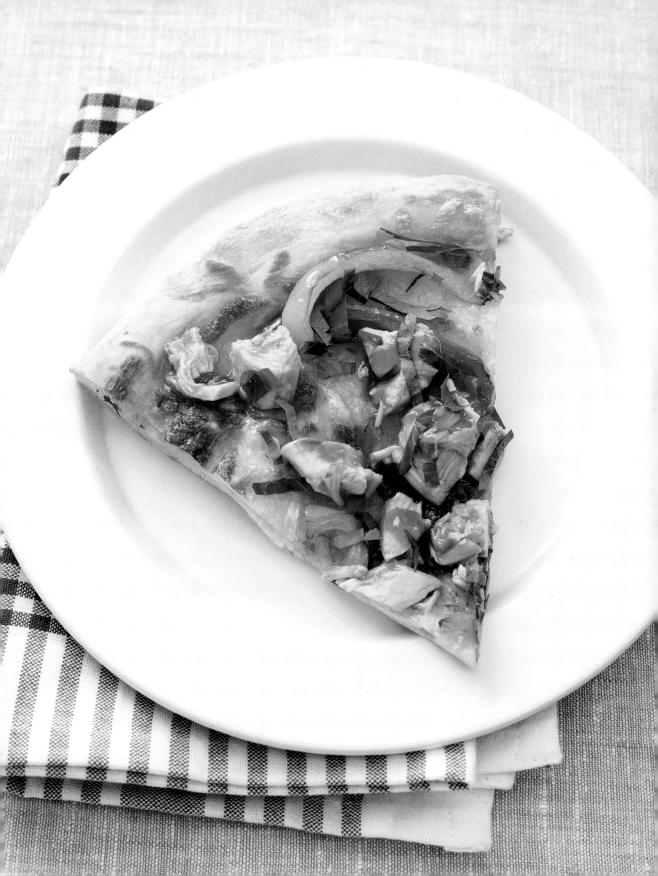

Cat Cora's Prosciutto, Pear, and Blue Cheese Sushi

Prep: *20 minutes* | **Total time:** *20 minutes* | **Makes:** *4 servings*

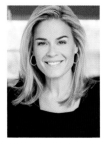

"Eating a balanced diet including complex carbohydrates such as brown rice keeps me going both in and out of the kitchen. This delicious, unique twist on sushi keeps me energized."

Cat Cora is the first and only female Iron Chef and author of *Cat Cora's Classics with a Twist* and *Cat Cora's Kitchen*. Cat Cora is also a busy mom of four young boys and the president and founder of the not-for-profit organization, Chefs for Humanity, whose mission is to reduce hunger worldwide.

3 cups cooked brown rice
4 tablespoons rice vinegar
½ teaspoon kosher salt
3 tablespoons pine nuts
4 sheets nori (seaweed)
4 slices prosciutto
2 tablespoons blue cheese
½ cup peeled, julienned pear
2 tablespoons balsamic glaze

1. Combine cooked rice, vinegar, and salt in a medium bowl; set aside. Toast and crush pine nuts; set aside.

2. Cover a sheet of aluminum foil with plastic wrap; top with 1 sheet nori. Press ¾ cup seasoned rice onto nori, leaving a ¼-inch border at the top and bottom. Press ½ tablespoon crushed pine nuts into the rice; top with 1 slice prosciutto, ½ tablespoon blue cheese, and 2 tablespoons pear.

3. Roll foil tightly toward you; remove foil and plastic wrap. Cut roll into 1-inch pieces with a sharp, wet knife.

4. Repeat steps with 3 more rolls. Drizzle pieces of each sushi roll evenly with 1½ teaspoons balsamic glaze.

Serving size: 1 roll Calories 280; Fat 8.4g (sat 1.9g, mono 2g, poly 2.7g); Cholesterol 14mg; Protein 11g; Carbohydrate 40g; Sugars 4g; Fiber 4g; Iron 1mg; RS 2.5g; Sodium 686mg

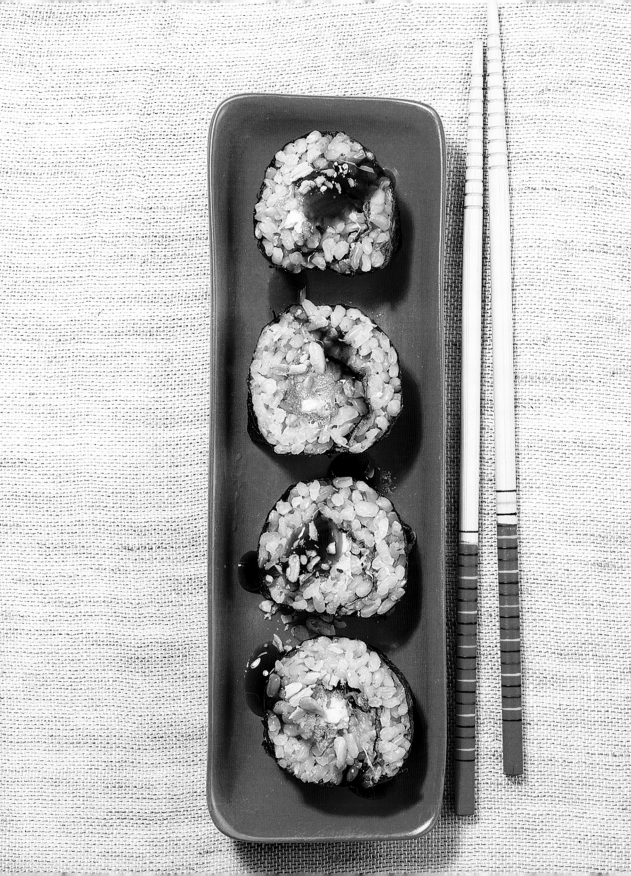

Carla Hall's Quick Chicken Mole

Prep: *5 minutes* | **Cook:** *20 minutes* | **Total time:** *25 minutes* | **Makes:** *6 servings*

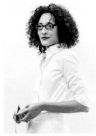

"Mole is the perfect solution for chocolate lovers to have chocolate before dessert, not to mention packing in the healthful antioxidants that chocolate possesses. Besides chicken, try the mole on beef, seasoned tofu, drizzled over rice and beans, and even as a condiment."

Carla Hall is the owner and executive chef of Alchemy Caterers in Washington, D.C., which features savory and sweet artisanal baked goods; she's also a co-host of ABC's *The Chew;* and a season-five finalist on Bravo's Top Chef.

1 tablespoon vegetable oil
1 medium onion, finely chopped
2 garlic cloves, minced
1½ teaspoons ground cumin
1 teaspoon ground cinnamon
½ teaspoon salt
¼ teaspoon freshly ground black pepper
1 (28-ounce) can diced tomatoes
1 (4-ounce) can diced green chiles
1 teaspoon tahini
3 ounces chopped dark chocolate
1 tablespoon chopped cilantro
1 rotisserie chicken, divided into 6 pieces, warmed
½ avocado, pitted and sliced
1 tomato, diced

1. Heat oil over medium heat in a large saucepan. Add onion; cook for 3 minutes or until translucent. Add garlic; cook for 1 minute. Stir in cumin, cinnamon, salt, and pepper; cook for 1 minute.

2. Add canned diced tomatoes and chiles to saucepan; simmer for 10 minutes. Stir in tahini and chocolate until melted. Stir in chopped cilantro; remove from heat and cool slightly. Process in a blender or food processor for 30 seconds or until smooth. (Add some water if sauce is too thick.) Spoon sauce over chicken. Serve with avocado and tomato.

Serving size: ⅙ chicken with sauce Calories 354; Fat 17.2g (sat 5.7g, mono 6.2g, poly 3.6g); Cholesterol 85mg; Protein 31g; Carbohydrate 19g; Sugars 11g; Fiber 5g; Iron 3mg; RS 0g; Sodium 648mg

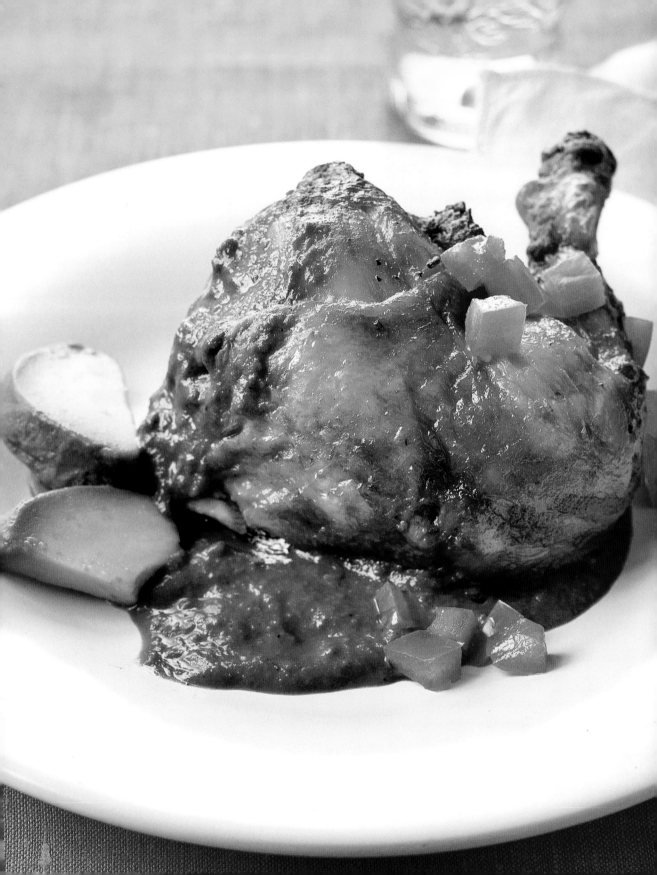

Michael Chiarello's Fusilli Michelangelo with Roasted Chicken

Prep: 10 minutes | *Cook:* 20 minutes | *Total time:* 30 minutes | *Makes:* 6 servings

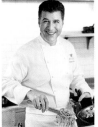

"This dish is one of my all-time favorites. It's tasty, simple, and full of flavor."

Michael Chiarello is the nationally renowned chef/owner of Bottega, his highly acclaimed Napa Valley restaurant in Yountville, California. An Emmy-winning Food Network host and *Top Chef Masters* finalist, Chiarello is also a winemaker and the tastemaker behind NapaStyle, a culinary retail store and catalog.

7	sun-dried tomatoes
1½	tablespoons balsamic vinegar
1½	teaspoons sugar
½	pound whole wheat fusilli
2	tablespoons olive oil
4	cups sliced mushrooms
2	minced garlic cloves
½	cup fresh basil
1½	cups tomato sauce
½	cup plus ⅓ cup grated Parmesan cheese
1	rotisserie chicken, meat removed (skin discarded)
3	cups arugula
2	tablespoons toasted pine nuts

1. Place sun-dried tomatoes in a bowl. Bring balsamic vinegar, sugar, and 3 tablespoons water to a boil. Pour over tomatoes; let stand 10 minutes. Drain and slice.

2. Cook pasta according to package directions; reserve ½ cup cooking water and drain.

3. Heat oil in a nonstick skillet over medium heat. Add mushrooms. Cook 1 minute without stirring, then cook, stirring, 5 minutes or until browned. Add garlic; cook 1 minute. Add basil and reserved tomatoes; cook 1 minute. Add tomato sauce; bring to a simmer. Add pasta, ½ cup grated Parmesan, reserved cooking water, chicken; toss, and transfer to serving bowl. Add arugula, pine nuts, and remaining Parmesan. Serve.

Serving size: 1⅓ cups Calories 431; Fat 16.9g (sat 4.6g, mono 7.2g, poly 3.4g); Cholesterol 81mg; Protein 37g; Carbohydrate 36g; Sugars 6g; Fiber 5g; Iron 4mg; RS 1.5g; Sodium 620mg

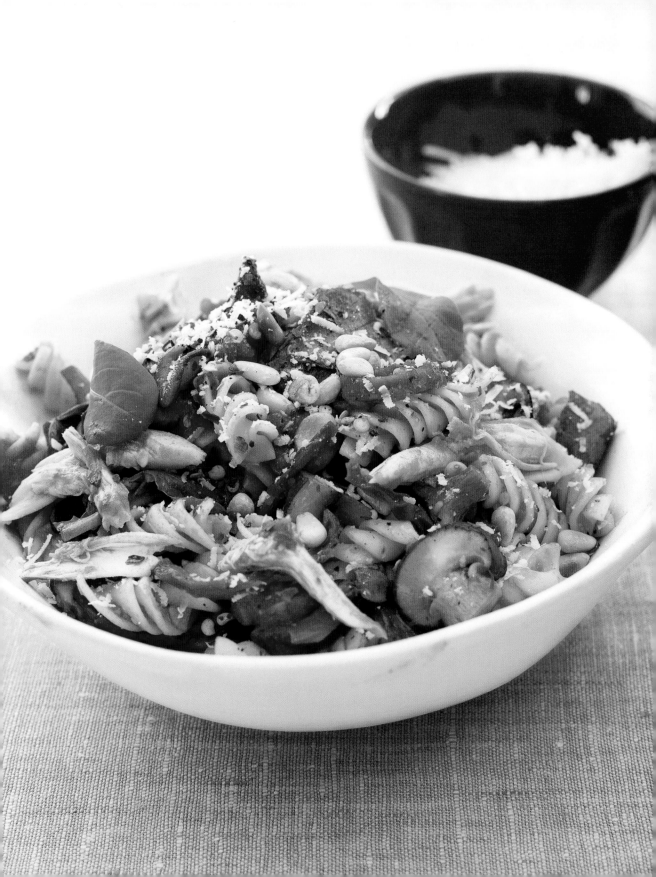

Donatella Arpaia's Edamame and Pear Crostini

Prep: 5 minutes | **Cook:** 20 minutes | **Total time:** 25 minutes | **Makes:** 10 servings

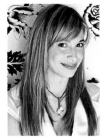

"Edamame and pear plays well on the traditional combination of fava beans and pear. It's healthy, sweet, and crunchy with great texture and flavor. This light appetizer is perfect for a baby or bridal shower."

Donatella Arpaia is the owner of Donatella, DBar, and Kefi in New York City; and a guest judge on Food Network's *Iron Chef America* and *The Next Iron Chef*. She is also a regular contributor on the *Today* show; and is the author of *Donatella Cooks: Simple Food Made Glamorous*.

1 (16-ounce) bag frozen shelled edamame
¼ cup extra virgin olive oil, divided
1 cup chopped fresh mint, plus additional for garnish
½ cup grated Pecorino Romano cheese
½ teaspoon salt
¼ teaspoon freshly ground black pepper
1 (12-ounce) baguette, thinly sliced
1–2 large Bartlett pears, peeled and diced

1. Preheat oven to 375°.

2. Cook edamame in salted boiling water for 10 minutes. Remove with a slotted spoon, and place in ice water; drain. Set aside ¼ cup whole edamame; process the remainder in a food processor until coarsely chopped. Combine mashed edamame with reserved whole edamame, 3 tablespoons oil, 1 cup mint, cheese, salt, and pepper.

3. Place baguette slices on a baking sheet, brush lightly with remaining 1 tablespoon oil, and bake for 10 minutes. Top each baguette slice with 1 tablespoon edamame mixture and 2 teaspoons pear. Garnish with additional mint, if desired.

Serving size: 3 crostini Calories 241; Fat 8.9g (sat 1.7g, mono 4.4g, poly 0.6g); Cholesterol 6mg; Protein 12g; Carbohydrate 29g; Sugars 2g; Fiber 4g; Iron 4mg; RS 0.6g; Sodium 445mg

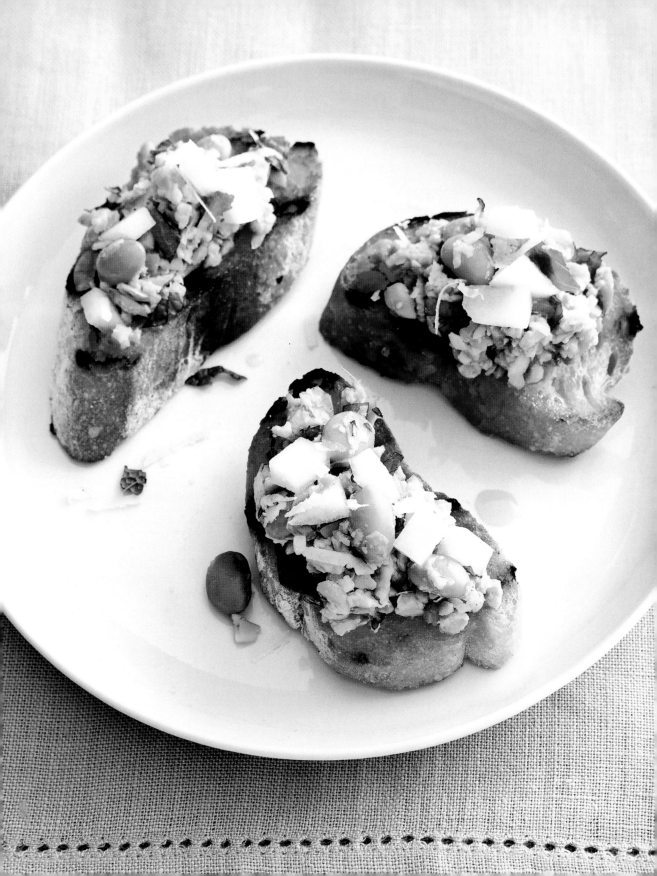

RS
1.2g

Emily Luchetti's Brown Rice Pudding

Prep: 2 minutes | *Cook:* 20 minutes (*plus 10–15 minutes cooling*) | *Total time:* 32 minutes | *Makes:* 4 servings

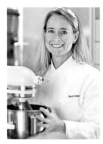

"I eat brown rice and veggies often for dinner. One night I had a sweet tooth, so I turned my leftover brown rice into a quick and not too unhealthy dessert. The nutty rice goes well with the juicy ripe fruit."

Emily Luchetti is the executive pastry chef at Farallon and Waterbar restaurants in San Francisco. She has won numerous awards, including the James Beard Foundation Outstanding Pastry Chef award, and is the author of six cookbooks. Her latest is *The Fearless Baker.*

2 cups low-fat (1%) milk
3 tablespoons brown sugar
2 cups cooked brown rice
2 tablespoons heavy cream
⅛ teaspoon salt
2 cups fresh stone fruit when in season (or 1 cup golden raisins, dried apricots, and/or sour cherries)

1. Combine milk and brown sugar in a medium saucepan. Briefly bring to a boil, whisking; reduce to a simmer. Cook, stirring occasionally, until liquid has reduced to 1½ cups, about 10 minutes.

2. Stir in rice and cook for 5–10 minutes, until some of the liquid has been absorbed. (There should still be some liquid in the pan; it will get firmer as it cools.)

3. Remove from heat and cool to room temperature. Stir in cream and salt.

4. Serve in bowls with fruit on top. (You can refrigerate the rice pudding overnight. If it is too thick for your liking the next day, whisk in a little milk.)

Serving size: ½ cup rice pudding and ½ cup fresh fruit or ¼ cup dried fruit Calories 223; Fat 3.3g (sat 1.8g, mono 1g, poly 0.3g); Cholesterol 11mg; Protein 5g; Carbohydrate 44g; Sugars 23g; Fiber 4g; Iron 1mg; RS 1.2g; Sodium 93mg

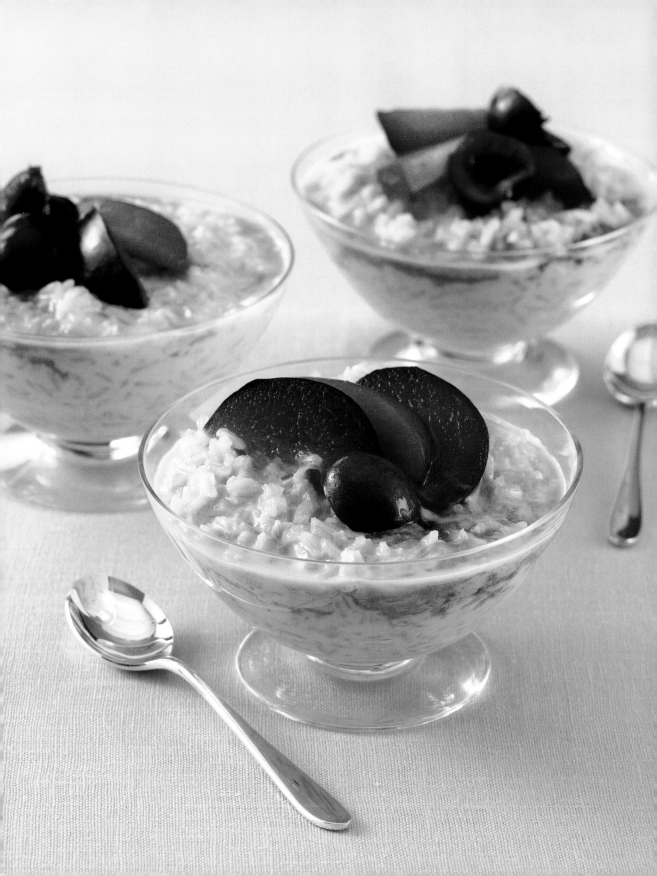

RS
3.7g

Candice Kumai's Pearl Barley with Peas and Edamame

Prep: *5 minutes* | **Cook:** *30 minutes* | **Total Time:** *35 minutes* | **Makes:** *4 servings*

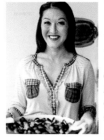

"Carbs are the ultimate food in my book. I will never—mark my words—cut them from my diet! My day is filled with them, from my morning muesli to a late-night pizza with the girls."

Candice Kumai is a healthy-lifestyle chef, author, and television host. She is the author of *Pretty Delicious: Lean and Lovely Recipes for a Healthy, Happy New You*, a guest judge on *Iron Chef America*, co-host of Lifetime television's hit series *Cook Yourself Thin*, chef contributor on Cooking Channel's *Unique Eats*, and an alum of *Top Chef*.

1	cup dry pearl barley
1	cup shelled frozen edamame
1	cup frozen peas
1	cup fresh spinach, chopped
2¼	teaspoons Worcestershire sauce
1½	teaspoons lemon zest
1½	tablespoons fresh lemon juice
¼	teaspoon sea salt

1. Place barley and 4 cups water in a medium saucepan; bring to a boil. Cover, reduce heat to low, and cook until water is nearly absorbed, 25–30 minutes. Stir in edamame and peas and cook, uncovered, until barley absorbs all of the remaining water, 5–10 minutes. Remove from heat.

2. Stir in spinach; set aside. Combine Worcestershire sauce, lemon zest, lemon juice, and sea salt in a small bowl, whisking well. Pour vinaigrette over barley; stir to combine. Serve warm or at room temperature.

Serving size: About 1 cup Calories 227; Fat 2.4g (sat 0.3g, mono 0.6g, poly 1.1g); Cholesterol 0mg; Protein 10g; Carbohydrate 43g; Sugars 4g; Fiber 9g; Iron 4mg; RS 3.7g; Sodium 213mg

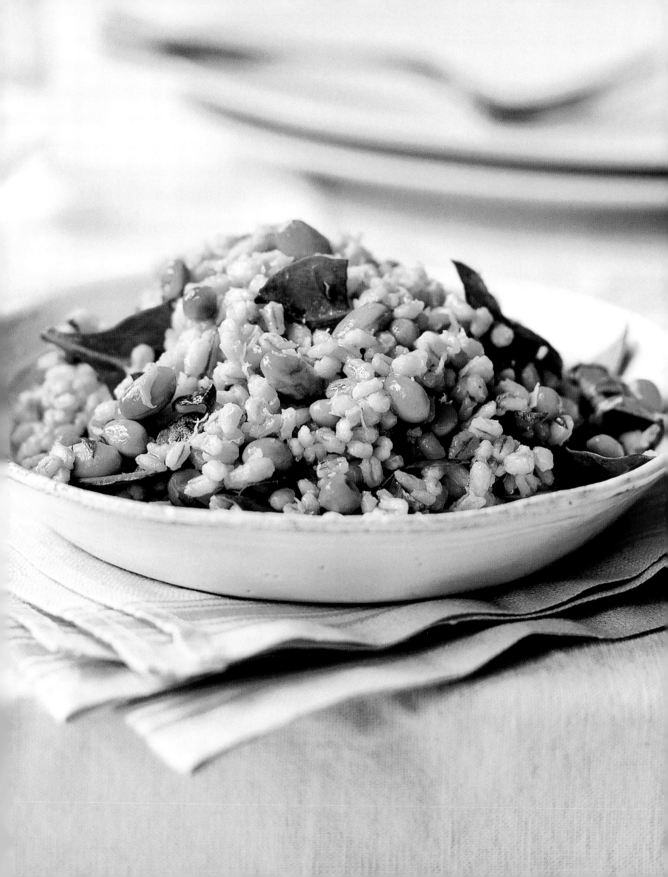

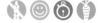

Cristina Ferrare's Grilled Polenta Cakes

Prep: 5 minutes | **Cook:** 31 minutes | **Total Time:** 36 minutes | **Makes:** 10 servings

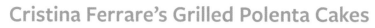

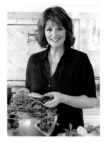

"I keep ready-made polenta on hand for when I need a quick appetizer. I enjoy grilled polenta cakes plain or with a tomato bruschetta topping, brushed with pesto, or with a simple tomato sauce, like this recipe."

Cristina Ferrare is a *New York Times* best-selling author and host of her own cooking show, *Cristina Ferrare's Big Bowl of Love*, on OWN (the Oprah Winfrey Network). She has a home decor company, Ferrare with Company, and a retail shop, Marquette Home.

1   (18-ounce) tube polenta
¼   cup extra virgin olive oil
    Cooking spray
1   cup of your favorite tomato sauce
½   cup freshly shredded Parmesan cheese (you may have some left over)
¼   cup whole basil leaves
    Pinch of kosher salt
⅛   teaspoon freshly ground black pepper

1. Remove polenta from casing, cut into ten ½-inch slices (cakes), and pat dry with paper towels.

2. Brush both sides of polenta cakes with oil, and set aside.

3. Heat a grill pan over high heat until hot. Lay polenta cakes in one layer on the pan; grill for 8–10 minutes on each side or until both sides are golden and crunchy and have grill marks.

4. Remove cakes from the grill pan and let cool on a wire rack. Preheat the oven to 350°.

5. Coat a baking sheet with cooking spray. Arrange the grilled polenta cakes on the baking sheet. Place 1 tablespoon of tomato sauce on each slice, then add 1–2 teaspoons Parmesan to each. Bake for 15 minutes.

6. Garnish with basil, salt, and pepper. Serve warm.

Serving size: 1 cake Calories 116; Fat 7g (sat 1.5g, mono 4.6g, poly 0.7g); Cholesterol 4mg; Protein 3g; Carbohydrate 10g; Sugars 1g; Fiber 1g; Iron 0mg; RS 0.3g; Sodium 387mg;

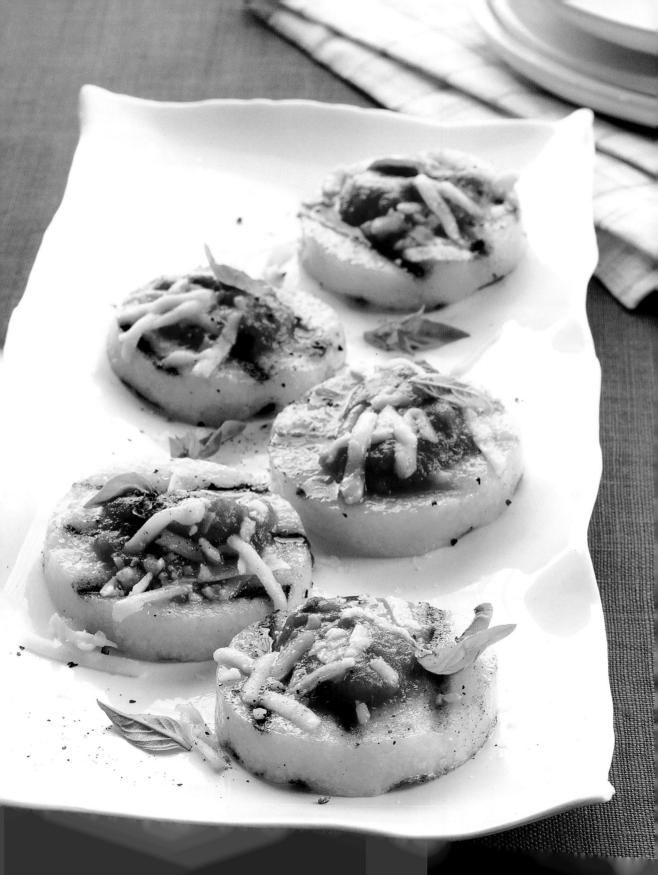

RS
2g

Joe Bastianich's Scoglio (Seafood Pasta)

Prep: *5 minutes* | **Cook:** *47 minutes* | **Total Time:** *52 minutes* | **Makes:** *6 servings*

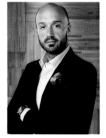

"Carbs—especially pasta—are the fuel my body needs to maintain an athletic lifestyle. This classic Italian dish, loaded with delicious iron-rich shellfish, is both sustaining and satisfying."

Joe Bastianich is a famed restaurateur, winemaker, author, and television personality. Bastianich is a judge on the hit FOX series *MasterChef* and *MasterChef Italia* in Italy. His newest book, *Restaurant Man,* is due to be released in spring 2012.

FOR SAUCE:

- 2 tablespoons olive oil
- 2 garlic cloves, crushed
- 1 (16-ounce) can whole Italian tomatoes
  Salt and freshly ground black pepper, to taste
- 1 teaspoon Sicilian oregano (optional)

FOR PASTA:

- 1 pound dry spaghetti
- 2 tablespoons plus 2 teaspoons olive oil, divided
- 4–6 medium-size scallops
- ¼ teaspoon salt
- ¼ teaspoon pepper
- 8 medium-size peeled shrimp
- 1 sprig fresh oregano
- 1 sprig fresh thyme
- 8 mussels
- 8 clams
- ½ cup white wine

MAKE SAUCE:

1. Heat oil in a saucepan over medium heat. Add garlic to oil and cook, stirring, until golden brown. While garlic browns, pour tomatoes into a bowl; break them up using clean hands. Once garlic is browned, add tomatoes and their juices. Add salt and pepper (and oregano if using).

2. Simmer over low heat for 45 minutes, adding water to keep the sauce from becoming too thick. The sauce should be a rich red color. If it turns brick red, it's too thick.

MAKE PASTA:

1. Cook pasta according to package directions. Drain, reserving 1 cup cooking water.

2. Heat 2 tablespoons oil in a large skillet. Season scallops with salt and pepper; cook over medium high heat, about 2–3 minutes per side, until golden brown on each side. Remove and set aside.

3. In the same pan, cook shrimp until they just turn pink, about 1–2 minutes. Remove and set aside.

4. Add reserved pasta water to pan along with oregano and thyme. Simmer for 10 minutes to

CONTINUED ON PAGE 282

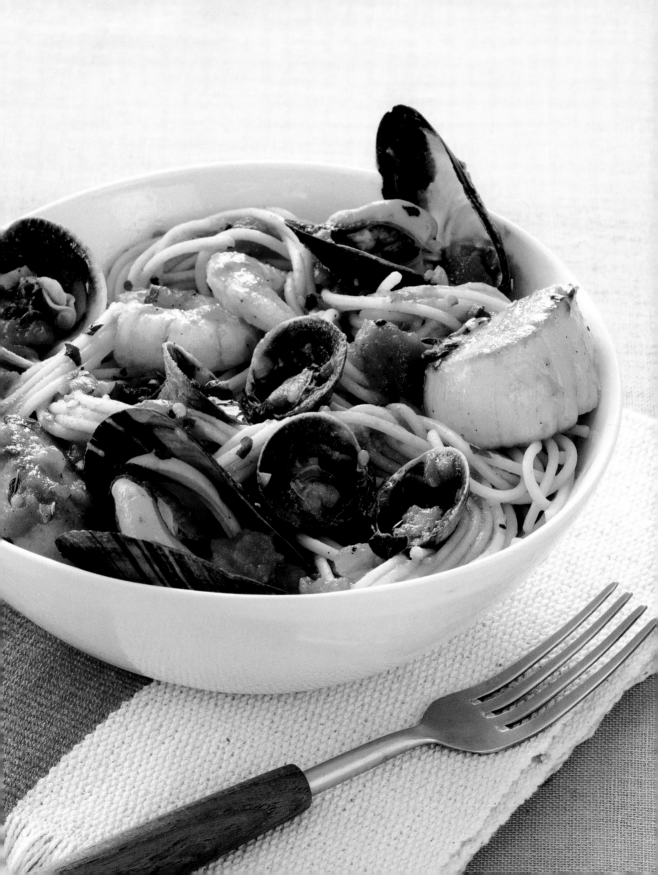

Joe Bastianich's Scoglio (Seafood Pasta)

create a fish broth, scraping the bottom of the pan with a spatula to release the caramelized bits left over from sautéing into the broth.

5. Once the broth is ready, add mussels with remaining 2 teaspoons oil and cover. Cook 2–3 minutes, removing mussels as soon as they open. Set aside. Repeat with the clams, cooking about 4 minutes. Remove and set aside.

6. Strain the remaining fish broth through a sieve and return to the same pan. Add wine and simmer over medium heat, 2–3 minutes, to burn off the alcohol. Add scallops back to the pan. Then add ½ cup pomodoro sauce. Add shrimp and a little more pomodoro sauce. Add pasta to the saucepan, stirring to coat with pomodoro sauce. Simmer 2–3 minutes and fold clams and mussels into the pasta. Serve immediately.

Serving size: about 2 cups Calories 433; Fat 10.4g (sat 1.6g, mono 6.1g, poly 1.6g); Cholesterol 25mg; Protein 19g; Carbohydrate 61g; Sugars 2g; Fiber 4g; Iron 4mg; RS 2g; Sodium 491mg

TIP:
Keep shellfish and fresh fish cold before you start cooking. Place in a bowl, cover with a damp towel, and let chill in the coldest part of the fridge.

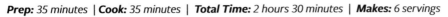

Gail Simmons's Individual Spinach and Mushroom Pizzas with Whole Wheat Crust

Prep: 35 minutes | **Cook:** 35 minutes | **Total Time:** 2 hours 30 minutes | **Makes:** 6 servings

RS
3.2g

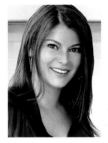

"Pizza is one of those foods I could never give up. The combination of crispy crust, tangy sauce, and fresh mozzarella is always so satisfying. I also love adding chile flakes before serving for a little extra little kick."

Gail Simmons is a celebrated culinary expert, food writer, and television personality who has worked in some of the country's most notable restaurants. The host of *Top Chef: Just Desserts*, Bravo's pastry-focused spin-off of the *Top Chef* franchise, she is also a judge on *Top Chef Masters*.

FOR CRUST:

- 1   packet active dry yeast
- 1   cup very warm water (100°–110°)
- ½   teaspoon sugar
- 1½ cups whole wheat flour
- 1½ cups unbleached all-purpose flour plus more for kneading
- 1   teaspoon fine sea salt
- ¼   cup olive oil

FOR TOPPINGS:

- 1   tablespoon olive oil, divided, plus more for drizzling (optional)
- 8   ounces cremini mushrooms, cleaned well and patted dry, thinly sliced
- 6   ounces baby spinach
     Pinch of coarse sea salt, plus more for sprinkling on top (optional)
- 1   (28-ounce) can whole tomatoes, juices drained
- 4   ounces fresh, salted mozzarella, thinly sliced
- 2   large garlic cloves, thinly sliced
     Crushed red pepper (optional)

MAKE CRUST:

1. Put yeast in a small bowl; add water and sugar. Gently whisk to combine. Let stand until foamy, about 5 minutes.

2. Mix together flours and salt in a large bowl. Form a well in center of flour. Pour oil into the well and, with clean hands, rub oil into flour. Add yeast mixture to flour; mix to combine. Knead dough on a lightly floured work surface until smooth and elastic, about 6 minutes. Form dough into a ball, place in an oiled bowl, cover with plastic wrap and a clean dish towel, and let dough rise at room temperature for 90 minutes.

3. About 30 minutes before dough is ready, preheat oven to 500° with rack in center and pizza stone on rack. Once the oven reaches temperature, heat stone for at least 30 minutes.

MAKE TOPPINGS:

1. Heat ½ tablespoon oil in a large skillet over medium-high heat. Add mushrooms; cook until tender, about 2 minutes. Transfer to a small colander set over a bowl to drain excess liquid. Add remaining oil to skillet, and add spinach; cook

CONTINUED ON PAGE 284

283

Gail Simmons's Individual Spinach and Mushroom Pizzas with Whole Wheat Crust

until wilted and deep green, about 2 minutes. Transfer to a plate. Place tomatoes in a bowl and, with clean hands, break up into small pieces. Season sauce with salt.

2. When dough is ready, gently remove from bowl and cut into 6 pieces. Work with 1 piece of dough at a time, keeping unused dough covered with plastic wrap. Using both hands, roll into a ball, then press into a flat round, about 4 inches in diameter. Using a floured rolling pin, roll out dough on a lightly floured surface to a 7-inch round; transfer to a floured pizza peel.

3. Spread about $\frac{1}{4}$ cup sauce onto dough, leaving a $\frac{1}{4}$-inch border at edge. Working quickly, sprinkle with some of garlic, then add $\frac{1}{6}$ of the mozzarella. Top with $\frac{1}{6}$ of the spinach and $\frac{1}{6}$ of the mushrooms. If desired, lightly drizzle pizza with additional oil and sprinkle with salt. Slide pizza off of peel onto stone and bake until edges are puffed and golden, about 5–6 minutes.

4. Transfer pizza to a cutting board; cut into 6 slices and serve immediately, with red pepper flakes, if desired. Repeat with remaining ingredients.

Serving size: 1 pizza Calories 418; Fat 16.1g (sat 3.3g, mono 5.6g, poly 0.9g); Cholesterol 15mg; Protein 14g; Carbohydrate 56g; Sugars 4g; Fiber 7g; Iron 5mg; RS 3.2g; Sodium 811mg;

> **TIP:**
> Make these pizzas a healthy, satisfying meal by adding a crisp green salad and a glass of red wine.

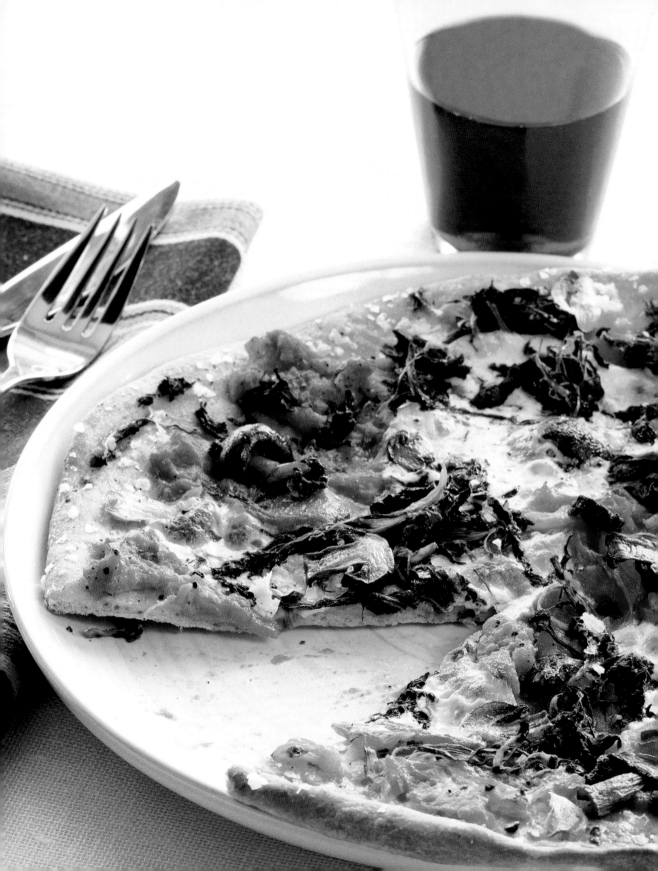

Allysa Torey's Date-Walnut Mini Cupcakes with Orange Cream Cheese Frosting

Prep: *20 minutes* | **Cook:** *15 minutes + cooling* | **Total Time:** *1 hour 20 minutes* | **Makes:** *48 servings*

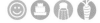

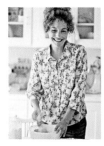

"The inspiration for this recipe came from my memories of sitting around the kitchen table with my mom as a child and eating date-nut bread with cream cheese. My kids absolutely love these!"

Allysa Torey opened Magnolia Bakery in New York's Greenwich Village in the summer of 1996. After ten successful years, she sold the business to spend more time with her growing family. She lives on a small farm in upstate New York with her two children, Wilson Henry and Audrey Jane, and spends her time cooking and writing.

FOR CUPCAKES:

Cooking spray
1½ cups coarsely chopped pitted dates
⅔ cup firmly packed light brown sugar
⅓ cup light unsulphured molasses
4 tablespoons unsalted butter
1 cup unbleached all-purpose flour
⅓ cup whole wheat pastry flour
1 teaspoon baking soda
½ teaspoon salt
1 large egg, lightly beaten, at room temperature
1 teaspoon pure vanilla extract
1 cup chopped walnuts

FOR FROSTING:

½ pound block-style cream cheese, softened
2 tablespoons unsalted butter, softened
1 cup powdered sugar, sifted
1 teaspoon freshly squeezed orange juice
½ teaspoon grated orange zest
½ teaspoon pure vanilla extract

GARNISH:

½ cup chopped walnuts

MAKE CUPCAKES:

1. Preheat oven to 350° and coat four 12-cup mini muffin tins with cooking spray.

2. Combine dates, brown sugar, molasses, butter, and 1 cup water in a medium saucepan over medium-high heat. Cover and bring to a boil. When mixture comes to a boil, remove from heat, transfer to a heatproof bowl, and allow to come to room temperature, about 45 minutes.

3. Combine flours, baking soda, and salt in a small bowl. Set aside.

4. When date mixture has cooled, place in a blender or food processor; process until smooth.

5. Transfer mixture to a large bowl. Add egg and vanilla; beat well. Add the dry ingredients in two parts; stir until incorporated, but do not overmix. Stir in the walnuts.

6. Carefully spoon batter into prepared cupcake tins, filling each cup about ¾ full. Bake for 10–12 minutes, or until a cake tester or knife inserted into center of cupcake comes out clean.

CONTINUED ON PAGE 288

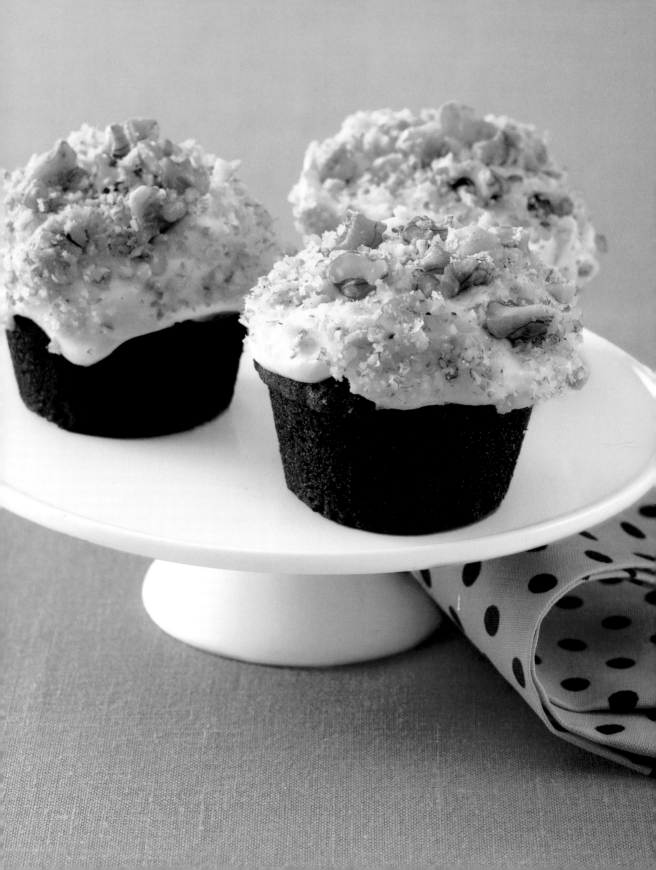

Allysa Torey's Date-Walnut Mini Cupcakes with Orange Cream Cheese Frosting

7. Cool cupcakes in the tins for 15 minutes. Remove from the tins and cool completely on a wire rack.

MAKE FROSTING:

1. Beat cream cheese and butter with an electric mixer on medium speed in a large bowl until smooth, about 3 minutes.

2. Add sugar, orange juice, orange zest, and vanilla; beat until creamy.

3. When cupcakes have cooled, decorate with frosting and sprinkle tops generously with walnuts. (Use frosting immediately, or cover and refrigerate for up to 2 hours, but no longer, before using.)

Serving size: 1 cupcake Calories 110; Fat 5.6g (sat 2.1g, mono 1.2g, poly 1.9g); Cholesterol 13mg; Protein 1g; Carbohydrate 14g; Sugars 10g; Fiber 1g; Iron 1mg; RS 0g; Sodium 69mg; Calcium 19mg

TIP:
If you're pressed for time, go ahead and use a lemon- or orange-flavored store-bought frosting on these yummy muffins.

Matt Lewis and Renato Poliafito's Holiday Sugar Cookies

Prep: *20 minutes* | **Cook:** *12 minutes* | **Chill:** *4 hours* | **Makes:** *24 (3-inch) cookies*

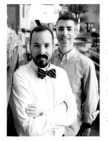

"For us, it is essential that sugar cookies taste as good as they look. Our whole wheat sugar cookies hold their shape well, and they have a wonderful nutty note via the whole wheat flour."

Co-owners of Baked, a New York City–based purveyor of outrageously delicious desserts made with the highest quality ingredients, Matt Lewis (right) and Renato Poliafito (left) are also the authors of two celebrated cookbooks, *Baked: New Frontiers in Baking*, and *Baked Explorations: Classic American Desserts Reinvented*.

FOR COOKIES:

- 1¼ cups all-purpose flour, plus more for rolling
- ¼ cup whole wheat flour
- ¼ teaspoon salt
- ½ teaspoon baking soda
- 4 ounces unsalted butter, softened
- ⅓ cup granulated sugar
- ⅓ cup light brown sugar
- 1 egg white
- 1¼ teaspoon pure vanilla extract
- ¼ teaspoon pure almond extract

FOR ICING:

- 2 cups powdered sugar, sifted
- ¼ cup pasteurized egg whites
- 2 teaspoons fresh lemon juice

MAKE COOKIES:

1. Preheat oven to 325°. Line 2 baking sheets with parchment paper and set aside.

2. Whisk together flours, salt, and baking soda in a medium bowl.

3. Beat butter and sugars together in a separate medium bowl with an electric mixer until light and fluffy. Scrape down sides and bottom of bowl. Add egg white and extracts; beat until just combined. Add flour mixture; stir until incorporated. Cover bowl with plastic wrap, and chill for at least 4 hours.

4. Dust a work surface with flour. Turn out chilled dough directly onto work surface. Roll dough out to a ¼-inch thickness. Use cookie cutters to cut shapes in dough, and gently transfer them to baking sheets. (You can reroll the scraps, just be sure to chill in between.)

5. Bake cookies for 12 minutes or until set but not browned. Remove cookies from oven, and cool for 5 minutes. Transfer cookies to a wire rack to cool completely.

CONTINUED ON PAGE 290

Matt Lewis and Renato Poliafito's Holiday Sugar Cookies

MAKE ICING:

1. Whisk together sugar, egg whites, and lemon juice in a large bowl until completely smooth. (If the icing is too thin, add a bit more sugar. If it's too thick, add a few more drops of lemon juice.)

2. Transfer icing to a pastry bag (or a resealable plastic bag with a small hole cut into one of the bottom corners). First, outline the cookie with icing, then fill it in, if desired. Let icing harden before serving. Cookies can be kept in an airtight container for up to 3 days.

Serving size: 1 cookie Calories 126; Fat 3.9g (sat 2.4g, mono 1g, poly 0.2g); Cholesterol 10mg; Protein 1g; Carbohydrate 22g; Sugars 16g; Fiber 0g; Iron 0mg; RS 0g; Sodium 59mg

TIP:
Don't stack your frosted and decorated cookies until they are completely dry, preferably overnight.

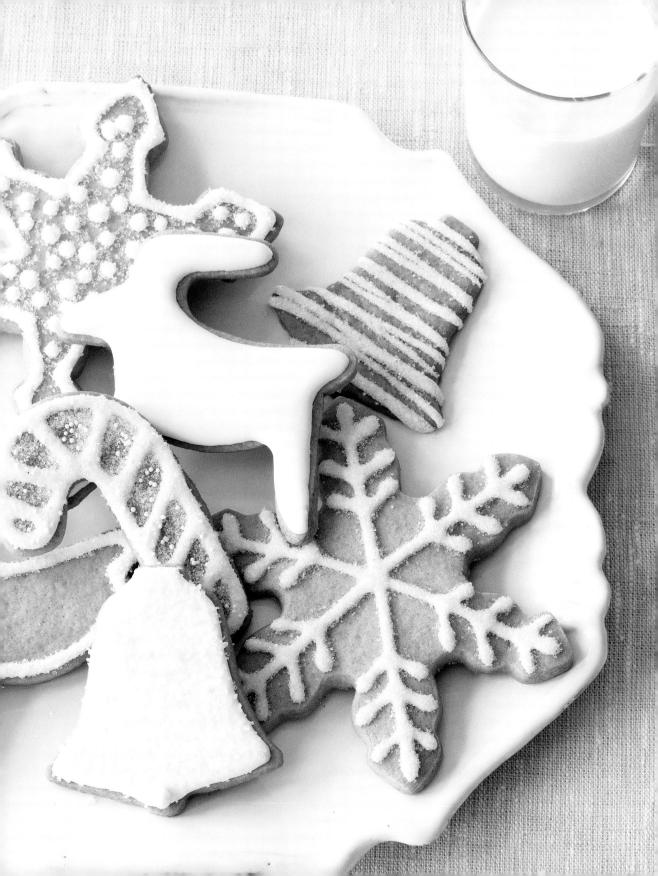

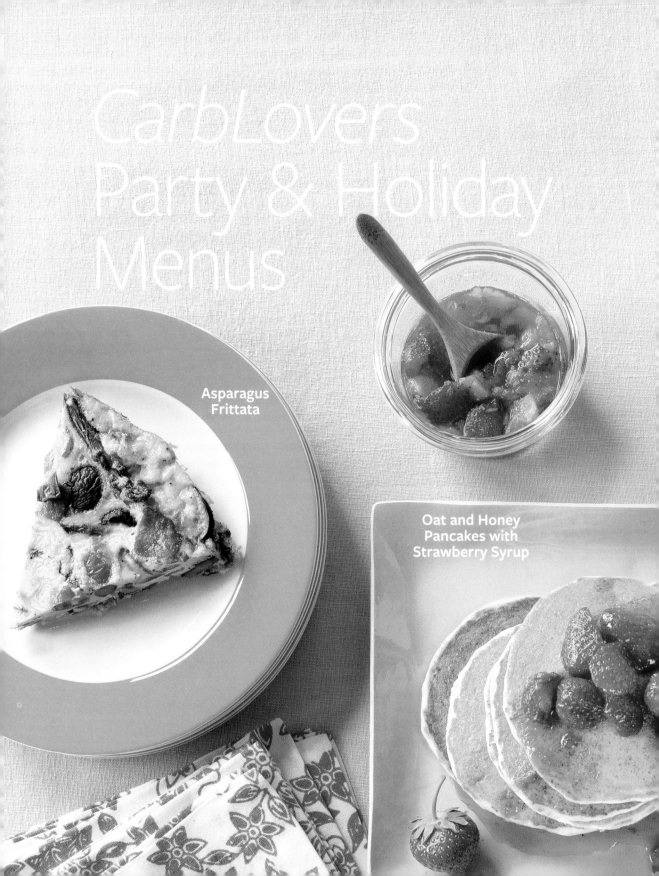

CarbLovers Party & Holiday Menus

Asparagus Frittata

Oat and Honey Pancakes with Strawberry Syrup

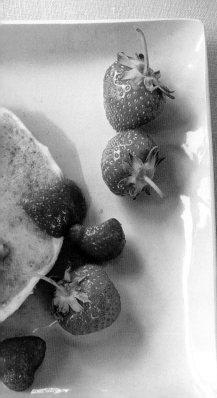

Peach Bellini

Fresh Citrus Salad

Think being on a diet and entertaining don't mix? We disagree! So we made sure the versatile and crowd-pleasing recipes in *The CarbLovers Diet Cookbook* were delicious enough to serve to guests. More important, we know from experience that it's a lot easier—and more fun—to lose weight while enjoying an active social life (saying no to party invitations and dinner with friends because you're afraid to overeat will just make you cranky . . . and even more vulnerable to bingeing). Our fun Game Day and Cocktail Party menus are the perfect blend of festive and filling, while our Spring Brunch, Romantic Dinner for Two, and Instant Weeknight Get-Together menus are as easy as they are elegant. We even included a yummy Kids Menu with foods they'll love—no need to tell 'em they're healthy!

Family Night Menu

With today's overscheduled families, it's often tough to get everyone to sit down together for dinner. Try setting aside at least one night a week to really connect with your family over a menu like this one.

STARTERS: Garbanzo Bean and Artichoke Bruschetta (page 218)

MAIN: Fresh Mozzarella, Basil, and Chicken-Sausage Pizza (page 136)

Green Salad with Vinaigrette [not in book]

DESSERT: Toasted Almond-Caramel Popcorn Clusters (page 250)

1. Make popcorn clusters.

2. Preheat oven to 475°. Make bruschetta and place on a platter for everyone to eat. Assemble salad in a large bowl, but do not add dressing.

3. Assemble and bake pizza. Dress salad. Remove pizza from oven; cool, slice, and serve.

4. Serve popcorn clusters for dessert.

Instant Weeknight Get-Together

Friends just told you they're in the neighborhood? Your mother-in-law invited herself over? No worries—this menu comes together in just 15 minutes!

DRINK: Beer

STARTER: Guacamole and Tortilla Chips [not in book]

MAIN: Shrimp Tacos with Lime Crema (page 148)

DESSERT: Bananas Foster (page 240)

1. An hour or so before guests arrive, pick up fresh guacamole and shrimp from the store (or use frozen shrimp that you have on hand). Buy beer if you'll be serving it.

2. Put beer in a large metal container with ice. When guests arrive, set out chips and guacamole, and let them serve themselves.

3. Make shrimp tacos and serve while hot.

4. Make dessert and enjoy with your guests!

Spring Brunch Menu

Whether you're celebrating Easter, Mother's Day, or a friend's new baby, spring always seems to bring lots of reasons to entertain. Our delicious menu has a little something for everyone and is gorgeous to boot.

COCKTAIL: Simple Peach Bellini (page 228)

STARTER: Fresh Citrus with Chopped Crystallized Ginger and Basil (page 40)

MAIN: Oat and Honey Pancakes with Strawberry Syrup (page 34)

Asparagus, Mushroom, and Tomato Frittata (page 46)

DESSERT: White Chocolate Banana Cream Pie (page 238)

1. Make pie from start to finish up to 1 hour before the party and reserve at room temperature. Or, if making the morning of the party, make it through step 2, cover surface of pudding with plastic wrap, and refrigerate. Add meringue before serving.

2. Make frittata an hour before guests arrive (or up to 1 day before). Reheat before serving.

3. Make citrus salad. Cover and refrigerate. Uncover 10 minutes before guests arrive.

4. About 20 minutes before guests arrive, make strawberry syrup for pancakes; set aside. Cook pancakes and stack on a foil-lined baking sheet. Keep warm in a 200° oven until ready to serve.

5. Pour everyone a bellini. Sit down with your guests and enjoy.

Summer Grilling Menu

When the weather starts warming up, we can't wait to fire up the grill. It's such a simple and fun way to entertain friends and family. Cleanup is minimal, so it's easy on you.

STARTERS: German Potato Salad (page 193)

Creamy Spinach-Artichoke Dip (page 222)

MAIN: Burgers 4 Ways: Asian, Tuscan, Southwestern, Provençale (page 160)

DESSERT: Oatmeal-Date-Chocolate Cookies (page 246)

Fresh Watermelon Slices

1. Make potato salad and cookies the day before your party.

2. The morning of, slice watermelon, transfer to a platter, cover with plastic wrap, and refrigerate. Also, make the dip and cover the surface directly with plastic wrap before refrigerating.

3. Decide which burgers you're going to make. Up to 3 hours before guests arrive, prep your patties. Place patties on a large plate or platter, cover with foil, and refrigerate. Prep any garnishes you'll be using for burgers.

4. About 20–30 minutes before guests arrive, preheat the grill. Remove potato salad and dip from fridge and bring to room temperature.

5. When guests arrive, start grilling!

Game Day Menu

Healthy food and sporting events don't usually go together, but our game-day eats are the exception. Of course, your guests don't need to know it's all good for them!

STARTERS: Layered Spicy Black Bean and Cheddar Dip (page 208)

Mexican Mole Chili (page 84)

Mini Corn and Feta Muffins (page 212)

MAIN: Bison Sliders with Guacamole (page 152)

DESSERT: Pecan Blondies (page 250)

1. Make chili and blondies the day before your party.

2. The morning of, bake muffins.

3. About an hour before company comes, make layered bean dip. Cover with plastic wrap and refrigerate until guests arrive. Prepare the patties for sliders, transfer to a large plate, cover with plastic wrap, and refrigerate.

4. Warm up chili, covered, on the stove over low heat (or in a slow cooker) about 30 minutes before quests arrive.

5. Preheat oven to 400°. Wrap muffins in foil; heat for 10–15 minutes before guests arrive.

6. Uncover dip and set out with a bowl of chips. Welcome your guests! While they snack on dip and chili, cook the sliders and make the guacamole. Serve hot.

Romantic Dinner for Two

Whether it's a first date or a night at home with your spouse, it's always fun to create a special meal for someone you love—and maybe stir up a little romance while you're at it! This menu is impressive *and* easy enough for you to focus on your company.

COCKTAIL: Simple Peach Bellini (page 228) or Champagne

STARTER: Edamame and Mushroom Potstickers (page 216)

MAIN: Spaghetti and Clams (page 116)

DESSERT: Mini Chocolate-Cinnamon Molten Cakes (page 242)

1. An hour or so before dinner, make the potstickers. Cover and refrigerate.

2. About 20 minutes before dinner, place a large pot of water on the stove to boil.

3. When your special guest arrives, pour him or her a bellini. Reheat potstickers in a frying pan over medium-high heat and place on a small serving plate, along with dipping sauce.

4. Assemble cakes in ramekins. Cover and refrigerate until ready to bake. Preheat oven to 350°.

5. Add pasta to boiling water and cook clams. Serve dinner.

6. Bring cakes to room temperature; bake.

Kids Menu

These recipes are a lot of fun and, most important, good for the kids—and you. Serve for a birthday party or sleepovers.

STARTER: Crispy Onion Rings (page 198)

MAIN: Individual Baked Mac and Cheese (page 118)

Cornflake-Crusted Chicken Tenders (page 168)

Steamed Broccoli with Parmesan [not in book]

DESSERT: Rocky Road Rice Crispy Treats (page 250)

1. Make rice crispy treats a day in advance. Cover with plastic wrap and store at room temperature.

2. Cook macaroni and assemble recipe in ramekins. Cover and refrigerate until ready to bake.

3. About 40 minutes before dinner, preheat oven to 400°. Bake ramekins.

3. Prepare and cook chicken tenders and keep warm.

4. Place the contents of a 10-ounce bag of frozen broccoli florets in a microwave-safe bowl. Microwave according to package directions; drain. Transfer to serving bowl and keep warm. Sprinkle with 2 tablespoons grated Parmesan before serving.

5. Make onion rings. Serve dinner. Enjoy dessert!

Winter Holiday Meal

Holiday entertaining can be stressful because you already have a million things to do, right? We keep it simple by using recipes that can be made ahead and reheated—without losing their fresh taste. Make it even easier by serving this meal buffet-style.

COCKTAIL: Mulled Cranberry Cocktail (page 228)

STARTER: Butternut Squash Soup (page 80)

MAIN: Roast Beef Tenderloin with Rosemary Roasted Potatoes (page 162)

DESSERT: Holiday Sugar Cookies (page 289)

Holiday Chocolate Bark (page 241)

1. Make cookies and chocolate bark up to a day in advance. Transfer to separate airtight containers. Great gift idea: Package up a little of each for guests to take home.

2. Make squash soup. Cool, cover, and refrigerate. An hour before the party, transfer soup to a slow cooker and heat to warm, or warm in a pot on the stovetop.

3. Up to 2 hours before guests arrive, make cranberry cocktail. Refrigerate or, if serving warm, keep on the stove over low heat.

4. About $1\frac{1}{2}$ hours before guests arrive, make roast beef with potatoes. Slice beef and arrange on platter with poatoes and some fresh rosemary.

5. Serve guests. Or if serving buffet-style, place all items on a large table or sideboard, and have guests help themselves.

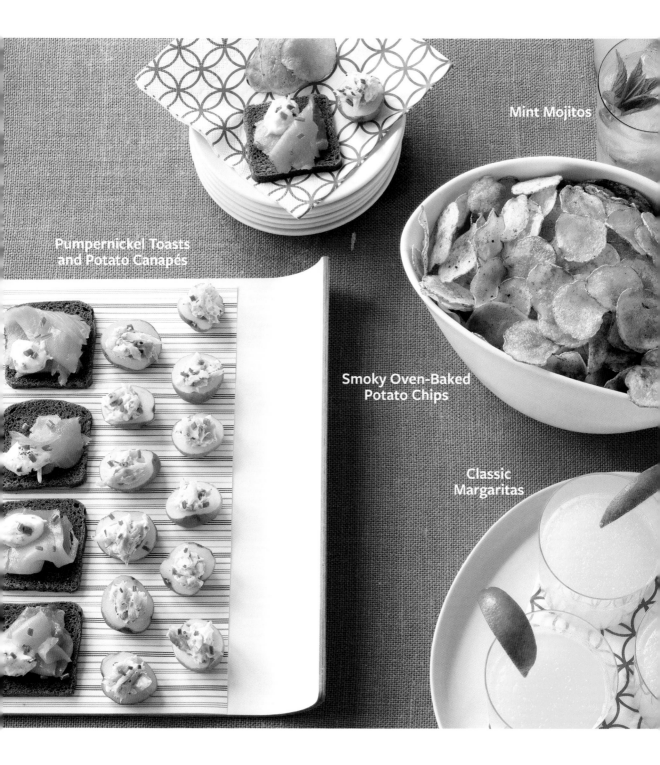

Mint Mojitos

Pumpernickel Toasts
and Potato Canapés

Smoky Oven-Baked
Potato Chips

Classic
Margaritas

CarbLovers Cocktail Party

Drinks and apps on a diet? Sure! Our light and delicious drinks and superslim bites will wow guests without weighing them down.

COCKTAILS: Mint Mojito, Classic Frozen Margarita (page 228)

APPETIZERS: Pumpernickel Toasts with Smoked Salmon and Lemon-Chive Cream (page 210)

Smoky Oven-Baked Potato Chips (page 214)

Potato Canapés Stuffed with Sour Cream and Smoked Trout (page 224)

DESSERT: Chocolate Brownie Bites (page 250)

1. Make potato chips the day before your party. Store in an airtight container. Bake brownie bites. Cover tightly with foil.

2. At least 3 hours before the party (or up to 2 days before), freeze the mixture for margaritas.

3. The day of, make canapés. Leave trout mixture (place, covered, in the refrigerator) off until ready to serve.

4. About 15 minutes before guests arrive, assemble pumpernickel toasts.

5. As guests arrive, blend margaritas and make mojitos. Have fun!

Book Club Menu

Don't get us wrong, we love our book club, but knowing that hosting duties are coming up always stresses us out. This menu—filled with totally doable recipes—will let you kick back and enjoy the conversation. And it's made up of recipes from Wolfgang Puck, Allysa Torey, and other celeb chefs, so you'll have even more to talk about!

DRINK: Your favorite bottles of red and white, plus sparkling water

STARTER: Edamame and Pear Crostini (page 272)

MAIN: Barbecue Chicken Pizza (page 264)

DESSERT: Date-Walnut Mini Cupcakes with Orange Cream Cheese Frosting (page 286)

1. Make cupcakes and frosting up to 2 hours before party. Frost right before guests arrive.

2. Grill or bake bread for crostini. Make edamame mixture. Assemble crostini about 10 minutes before guests arrive.

3. About 20 minutes before guests arrive, preheat oven to 500°. Assemble pizza. Welcome guests, and once the discussion gets going, place pizza in oven.

4. Open wine and serve.

5. When pizza is done baking, slice into wedges, or cut into bite-size pieces, depending on number of guests.

6. As the book talk is wrapping up, serve cupcakes.

PART 3
The *CarbLovers* Cookbook Diet Plan

The 7-Day *CarbLovers* Kickstart Meal Plan

This weeklong plan is the first phase of *The CarbLovers Diet*. It makes enjoying your favorite *CarbLovers* recipes—and losing up to 6 pounds—so easy and satisfying you won't believe you're dieting. These menus were carefully designed to satisfy your cravings for brain- and body-nourishing nutrients that keep you feeling full, while clocking in at about 1,200 calories a day. Feel free to mix and match any of these meals, but please move on to Phase 2 of the diet after seven days (you can always come back to the Kickstart if you start gaining). Oh, and don't even think about skipping a meal! The 7-Day *CarbLovers* Kickstart Meal Plan purposely includes breakfast, lunch, dinner, and one snack. You must stick to this pattern in order to maintain your energy and keep hunger at bay. Skipping just one meal might make you feel tired and stressed—and more likely to binge later. To keep it simple, every day we've included grab-and-go, and frozen options for dieters who are traveling or simply don't have time to cook. For even more no-cook options, go straight to page 316 for a list of *CarbLovers*-approved store-bought foods.

Day 1 Monday

BREAKFAST: Broiled Banana on Toast (page 52)

LUNCH: Black Bean, Avocado, Brown Rice, and Chicken Wrap (page 102)
OR
Lean Cuisine Ginger Garlic Stir Fry with Chicken

DINNER: Capellini with Bacon and Bread Crumbs (page 124)

SNACK: Rosemary and Garlic White Bean Dip (page 223) + ½ cup raw vegetables

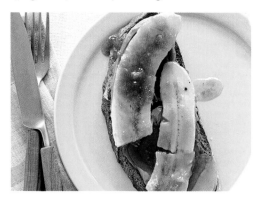

Day 2 Tuesday

BREAKFAST: Tropical Breeze Smoothie (page 66) + ½ medium slighty green banana

LUNCH: *CarbLovers* Club Sandwich (page 90)
OR
Amy's Kitchen Organic Medium Chili with Vegetables

DINNER: Shrimp Tacos with Lime Crema (page 148)

SNACK: 2 Laughing Cow Mini Babybel Light cheese wheels + 4 Wheat Thins or Triscuits

Day 3 Wednesday

BREAKFAST: Spinach and Egg Breakfast Wrap with Avocado and Pepper Jack Cheese (page 60)

LUNCH: Broccoli and Cheese–Stuffed Baked Potato (page 188)

DINNER: Creamy Barley Risotto with Peas and Pesto (page 127)
OR
Amy's Kitchen Mexican Casserole Bowl, light in sodium

SNACK: 10 baby carrots + 1 tablespoon low-fat ranch dressing

Day 4 Thursday

BREAKFAST: Banana Nut Oatmeal: Combine ½ cup old-fashioned rolled oats and 1 cup water in a small bowl. Microwave on high for 3 minutes. Top with one sliced banana, 1 tablespoon walnuts, 1 teaspoon cinnamon.

LUNCH: Roast Beef Pumpernickel Sandwich with Roasted Red Pepper, Arugula, and Goat Cheese (page 98)

DINNER: Grilled Chicken Cutlet with Summer Succotash (page 166) + side of whole wheat angel-hair pasta (1 cup) drizzled with 1 teaspoon extra virgin olive oil
OR
Healthy Choice Top Chef Café Steamers Grilled Chicken Pesto with Vegetables

SNACK: Toasted Almond-Caramel Popcorn Cluster (page 250)

Day 5 **Friday**

BREAKFAST: Tartine with Blackberry Thyme Salad (page 56) + 6-ounce low-fat yogurt

LUNCH: Barley Salad with Corn, Feta, Basil, and Charred Tomatoes (page 176) + 6 Wasa Crisp'n Light Mild Rye crispbread crackers
OR
Healthy Choice Top Chef Café Steamers Grilled Vegetables Mediterranean

DINNER: Maple-Glazed Cod with Baby Bok Choy (page 144) + ½ cup cooked brown rice Edamame and Mushroom Potstickers (page 216)

SNACK: White Bean and Herb Hummus with crudités: Mash ¼ can rinsed and drained white beans, 1 tablespoon chopped chives, 1 tablespoon lemon juice and 2 teaspoons olive oil. Enjoy with ½ cup fresh vegetables.

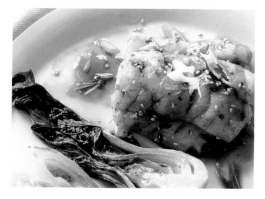

Day 6 **Saturday**

BREAKFAST: Steel-Cut Oatmeal with Salted Caramel Topping (page 38)

LUNCH: Stacked Deli Sandwich with Homemade Coleslaw (page 92)
OR
Lean Pockets Whole Grain Turkey, Broccoli & Cheese + 2 cups salad greens and ½ cup fat-free dressing

DINNER: Grilled Spice-Rubbed Pork Loin with Broccoli Rabe (page 151)

SNACK: Medium (slightly green) banana

Day 7 **Sunday**

BREAKFAST: Oat and Honey Pancakes with Smashed Strawberries (page 34) + 8 ounces 1% milk

LUNCH: Salmon Waldorf Salad (page 184) + 4 Wasa Crisp'n and Light Mild Rye crispbread crackers

DINNER: Pasta Primavera (page 112)
OR
Kashi Sweet & Sour Chicken

SNACK: Trail Mix: Combine ½ cup cornflakes, 2 tablespoons sliced almonds, and 2 tablespoons dried cherries.

> **TIP:**
> Love oatmeal? This is the plan for you! Our Banana Nut Oatmeal is the perfect go-to breakfast every day.

The 21-Day *CarbLovers* Immersion Meal Plan

By now you're probably eating and cooking healthier and have lost about 6 pounds. You're slimmer, happier, and ready for the next phase of *CarbLovers*. Boy, are you in for a treat! The 21-Day *CarbLovers* Immersion Meal Plan features bigger portions, more snacks (including cocktails!), more grab-and-go options, and even more delicious, indulgent recipes you can make yourself (think Buckwheat Crepes with Orange-Ricotta Filling for breakfast and Mini Chocolate-Cinnamon Molten Cakes for dessert!), as you eat about 1,600 calories a day. Just remember, you can mix and match any meal, even going back to the Phase 1 options if you like.

Your goal for the next three weeks is to lose about 2 pounds a week. By the end of Phase 2, many dieters will have lost 12 pounds or even more. If you still have more weight to lose, stick with the plan, returning to Phase 1 if you start to gain again. If you've met your weight-loss goal, congratulations! You can allow yourself a little more leeway when it comes to indulgences and eating out in restaurants. The dietitians who created *The CarbLovers Diet* have made sure that the newly slim you will stay that way as long as you stick to the *CarbLovers* way of eating.

WEEK 1

Day 1 Monday

BREAKFAST: Broiled Banana on Toast (page 52)

LUNCH: CarbLovers Club Sandwich (page 90) + Baked Lay's potato chips (1⅛-ounce bag)
OR
Lean Pockets Whole Grain Turkey, Broccoli & Cheese + Lärabar Cherry Pie mini bar

DINNER: Penne with Sausage and Spinach (page 134)

SNACK 1: Coffee-Vanilla Smoothie (8-ounce serving; page 66)

SNACK 2: Toasted Almond-Caramel Popcorn Clusters (page 250)

Day 2 Tuesday

BREAKFAST: Cornflakes with milk and berries: 2 cups cornflakes, 1 cup 1% low fat milk + 1 cup berries

LUNCH: Three Bean Soup with Canadian Bacon (page 72) + 1 whole-wheat roll

DINNER: Grilled Chicken Cutlet with Summer Succotash (page 166) + 2 cups salad greens and 2 tablespoons low-fat dressing
OR
Kashi Mayan Harvest Bake + 2 cups salad greens and 2 tablespoons low-fat dressing

SNACK 1: Rosemary and Garlic White Bean Dip (page 223) + 1 ounce pita chips

SNACK 2: 2 Oatmeal-Date-Chocolate Cookies (page 246)

Day 3 Wednesday

BREAKFAST: Banana-Nut Oatmeal: Combine ½ cup old-fashioned rolled oats + 1 cup water; microwave on high 3 minutes. Top with 1 sliced banana + 1 tablespoon chopped walnuts + 1 tablespoon cinnamon. Serve with 8-ounce glass of 1% milk.

LUNCH: Teriyaki Steak Sandwich (page 96) + medium apple
OR
Lean Pockets Whole Grain Culinary Creations Chipotle Chicken + piece of fruit

DINNER: Sausage, Tomato, White Bean, and Corkscrew Pasta Toss (page 120)

SNACK 1: Cup of fat-free or low-fat Greek yogurt, plain or with fruit

SNACK 2: 5-ounce glass of wine

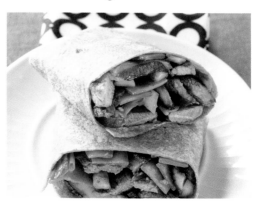

TIP:
Tell the world you're on a diet:
OK, maybe not everyone, but
letting a few close friends know
will help keep you motivated.

Day 4 **Thursday**

BREAKFAST: Chocolate-Antioxidant Boost Smoothie (page 66)

LUNCH: Grilled Cheese and Tomato on Rye (page 106) + Barley Salad with Corn, Feta, Basil, and Charred Tomatoes (page 176)

DINNER: Penne with Grilled Chicken and Vodka Sauce (page 121)
OR
Kashi Southwest Style Chicken + 2 cups salad greens and 2 tablespoons low-fat dressing

SNACK 1: Trail mix: Combine ½ cup cornflakes, 2 tablespoons sliced almonds, and 2 tablespoons dried cherries.

SNACK 2: Roasted Red Pepper and Zucchini Spread (page 220) + 3 baguette slices

Day 5 **Friday**

BREAKFAST: Broiled Banana on Toast (page 52)

LUNCH: Falafel Pita with Tahini Sauce (page 94)

DINNER: Creamy Barley Risotto with Peas and Pesto (page 127) + 2 cups mixed greens + 2 tablespoons low-fat dressing
OR
Amy's Kitchen Light & Lean Spinach Lasagna + 2 cups mixed greens + 2 tablespoons low-fat dressing

SNACK 1: Smoky Oven-Baked Potato Chips (11 chips; page 214)

SNACK 2: 5-ounce glass of wine

Day 6 **Saturday**

BREAKFAST: Oat and Honey Pancakes with Strawberry Syrup (page 34) + 6 ounces 1% low-fat milk

LUNCH: Creamy Cobb Salad (page 182) + Roasted Red Pepper and Zucchini Spread (page 220) + 3 slices baguette
OR
Dr. Praeger's California Veggie Burger + 2 slices whole-grain bread

DINNER: Mexican Mole Chili (page 84) with 2 Mini Corn and Feta Muffins (page 212)

SNACK 1: Chocolate Brownie Bite (page 250)

SNACK 2: 12-ounce light beer

Day 7 **Sunday**

BREAKFAST: Oatmeal-Cranberry Muffin (page 63)

LUNCH: Pan Bagnat (page 109)

DINNER: Spaghetti and Turkey Meatballs with Tomato Sauce + 2 cups mixed greens + 2 tablespoons low-fat dressing
OR
Amy's Kitchen Baked Ziti Bowl + 2 cups mixed greens + 2 tablespoons low-fat dressing

SNACK 1: Antipasto platter: 12 black olives + ½ cup bottled marinated artichoke hearts, drained, + ½ of a jarred roasted red bell pepper, sliced

SNACK 2: Banana "Ice Cream": Place 2 small frozen, sliced bananas + 6 tablespoons 1% low-fat milk in a blender or food processor and process until thick. Top with 2 tablespoons chopped walnuts.

WEEK 2

Day 8 Monday

BREAKFAST: Oatmeal-Cranberry Muffin (from batch that was made on Sunday) + Banana Shake: In a blender, combine 1 banana + 1½ cups 1% low-fat milk + ½ cup ice and blend.

LUNCH: Grilled Chicken Caesar with Pumpernickel Croutons (page 183)

DINNER: Grilled Flank Steak Fajitas (page 154)
OR
Ethnic Gourmet Chicken Korma

SNACK 1: 8 baked tortilla chips + ½ cup black beans mixed with ½ cup salsa

SNACK 2: Classic Frozen Margarita (page 228)

Day 9 Tuesday

BREAKFAST: Broiled Banana on Toast (page 52)

LUNCH: Hoppin' John (page 202) and 1 cup cooked quinoa
OR
Healthy Choice Café Steamers Grilled Basil Chicken + 2 cups mixed greens + 2 tablespoons low-fat dressing

DINNER: Spaghetti and Clams (page 116) + 2 cups mixed greens + 2 tablespoons low-fat dressing

SNACK 1: 1 ounce Brie + 1 small apple

SNACK 2: 4 Hershey's Kisses Special Dark Mildly Sweet Chocolates

Day 10 Wednesday

BREAKFAST: Peanut Butter–Banana Blast Smoothie (page 66)

LUNCH: Curried Tuna Salad Sandwich (page 93)

DINNER: Tortilla Chicken Soup (page 82)
OR
Ethnic Gourmet Pad Thai with Tofu

SNACK 1: 2 tablespoons store-bought hummus and 10 baby carrots

SNACK 2: 12-ounce light beer

Day 11 Thursday

BREAKFAST: Steel-Cut Oatmeal with Salted Caramel Topping (page 38) + green tea

LUNCH: Roasted Corn and Black Bean Burrito (page 104) + Campbell's Chunky Healthy Request Vegetable (1 cup)

DINNER: Fried Brown Rice with Edamame (page 200) + Edamame and Mushroom Potstickers (page 216)

SNACK 1: Granola with Pecans, Pumpkin Seeds, and Dried Mango (page 44)

SNACK 2: 6 ounces low-fat vanilla yogurt

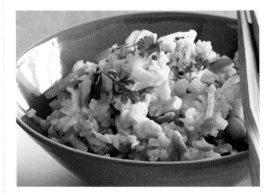

Day 12 Friday

BREAKFAST: Oat and Honey Pancakes with Strawberry Syrup (page 34)

LUNCH: Berry-Kale Smoothie (page 68) + 2 tablespoons store-bought hummus + one 6-inch pita

DINNER: Cornmeal Crusted Tilapia with Sautéed Greens and Whipped Honey Yams (page 146)
OR
Amy's Kitchen Mexican Casserole Bowl, light in sodium

SNACK 1: 12-ounce low-fat latte

SNACK 2: Chocolate Brownie Bite (page 250)

Day 13 Saturday

BREAKFAST: Eggs Benedict Florentine (page 36)

LUNCH: Roast Beef Pumpernickel Sandwich with Roasted Red Pepper, Arugula, and Goat Cheese (page 98)
OR
Progresso High Fiber Three-Bean Chili with Beef + 1 Laughing Cow Mini Babybel Original cheese + 3 Triscuit Original Crackers

DINNER: Fresh Mozzarella, Basil, and Chicken Sausage Pizza (page 136)

SNACK 1: Granola with Pecans, Pumpkin Seeds, and Dried Mango (page 44) + 12-ounce skim latte

SNACK 2: 5-ounce glass of wine

Day 14 Sunday

BREAKFAST: Asparagus, Mushroom, and Tomato Frittata (page 46) + 8 ounces orange juice

LUNCH: Barley Salad with Corn, Feta, Basil, and Charred Tomatoes (page 176) + 6 Wasa Crisp'n and Light Mild Rye crispbread crackers

DINNER: Orange Chicken Stir-Fry (page 172)
OR
Kashi Black Bean Mango

SNACK 1: 1 medium banana + 2 tablespoons almond butter

SNACK 2: Rosemary and Garlic White Bean Dip with 1 ounce pita chips (page 223)

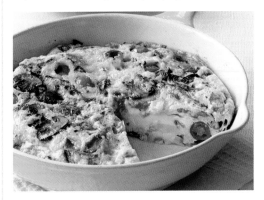

> **TIP:**
> Sip smarter with the delicious, super-slimming *CarbLovers* Fat-Flushing Cocktail (page 28).

The 21–DAY CARBLOVERS IMMERSION PLAN

Day 15 **Monday**

BREAKFAST: 2 cups cornflakes + 8 ounces 1% milk + 1 cup berries

LUNCH: Tuna and White Bean Crostino (page 100) + 1 cup Amy's Kitchen Organic Lentil Soup
OR
Guiltless Gourmet California Veggie Wrap + Newman's Own Organics Spelt Pretzels

DINNER: Capellini with Bacon and Bread Crumbs (page 124)

SNACK 1: Fat-free or low-fat Greek yogurt, plain or with fruit

SNACK 2: 3 cups air-popped popcorn

Day 16 **Tuesday**

BREAKFAST: Double Berry Smoothie (page 66)

LUNCH: Stacked Deli Sandwich with Homemade Coleslaw (page 92)

DINNER: Penne with Sausage and Spinach (page 134)
OR
Ethnic Gourmet Chicken Korma + 2 cups mixed greens + 2 tablespoons low-fat dressing

SNACK 1: Trail mix: Combine ½ cup cornflakes + 2 tablespoons sliced almonds + 2 tablespoons dried cherries

SNACK 2: 3 Hershey's Special Dark Miniatures

Day 17 **Wednesday**

BREAKFAST: Tartine with Blackberry Thyme Salad (page 56) + 6 ounce grapefruit or orange juice

LUNCH: Niçoise Salad (page 185) + 4 Wasa Crisp'n Light Mild Rye crispbread crackers or melba toast

DINNER: Mini Mediterranean Pizza (page 140)
OR
Healthy Choice Café Steamers Lemon Garlic Chicken and Shrimp + 2 cups mixed greens + 2 tablespoons low-fat dressing

SNACK 1: Medium banana + 2 tablespoons almond butter

SNACK 2: 2 Toasted Almond-Caramel Popcorn Clusters (page 250)

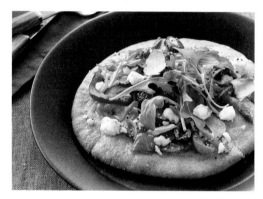

TIP:
Use fresh, in-season produce whenever possible. You'll get the most nutrients for your buck.

Day 18 **Thursday**

BREAKFAST: Banana-Nut Oatmeal: Combine ½ cup old–fashioned rolled oats + 1 cup water; microwave on high 3 minutes. Top with 1 sliced banana + 1 tablespoon chopped walnuts + 1 teaspoon cinnamon.

LUNCH: Chunky Tomato-Basil Soup with Pasta (page 76) + Grilled Cheese and Tomato on Rye (page 106)
OR
Evol Basic Bean & Cheese Burrito

DINNER: Gnocchi with Walnut-Arugula Pesto (page 128) + 2 cups salad greens + 2 tablespoons low-fat dressing

SNACK 1: Garbanzo Bean and Artichoke Bruschetta (4 pieces; page 218)

SNACK 2: 2 Oatmeal-Date-Chocolate Cookies (page 246)

Day 19 **Friday**

BREAKFAST: Banana-Nut Elvis Wrap (page 108) + 8 ounces 1% milk

LUNCH: Broccoli and Cheese–Stuffed Baked Potato (page 188)
OR
Progresso High Fiber Three-Bean Chili with Beef + Beanitos Black Bean chips

DINNER: Creamy Barley Risotto with Peas and Pesto (page 127) + 2 cups mixed greens + 2 tablespoons low-fat dressing

SNACK 1: Medium apple, pear, or 1 cup grapes + 8 Kashi TLC Crackers

SNACK 2: 5-ounce glass of wine

Day 20 **Saturday**

BREAKFAST: Huevos Rancheros (page 42)

LUNCH: Chicken Noodle Soup with Fall Vegetables (page 86)
OR
Evol Cilantro Lime Chicken Burrito

DINNER: Provençal Burger (page 160) + Sweet Potato Fries with Curried Ketchup (page 190)

SNACK 1: Medium slightly green banana

SNACK 2: Watermelon-Lime Granita (page 258)

Day 21 **Sunday**

BREAKFAST: Banana-Pecan Breakfast Bread (page 59) + ½ slightly green banana + Coffee-Vanilla Smoothie (8-ounce portion; page 66)
OR
Kashi Good Friends Cereal + ½ cup 1% milk + 2 Boca Breakfast Links

LUNCH: Black Bean, Avocado, Brown Rice, and Chicken Wrap (page 102)

DINNER: Ultimate Spinach and Turkey Lasagna (page 114) + 2 cups mixed greens + 2 tablespoons low-fat salad dressing

SNACK 1: Rosemary and Garlic White Bean Dip (page 223) with 1 ounce pita chips

SNACK 2: 5-ounce glass of wine

Grab and Go

We're all for you preparing your own delicious *CarbLovers* recipes from scratch, and even serving them on your best china by candlelight when the mood strikes. But we also know that's not always realistic. Sometimes you're just too busy, or too far from home, to even *think* about cooking. That's why we created this carefully curated list of *CarbLovers*-approved foods, which you can find at most major supermarkets or gourmet grocery stores. (For more, check out *The CarbLovers Diet Pocket Guide* or carblovers.com.) Our expert RDs screened each food to make sure it has the right components to be part of a *CarbLovers* weight-loss plan. Oh, and they taste good too (real dieters tried 'em all). So go ahead: Stock your freezer with frozen meals and your office drawers with cereal bars and snacks. As long as you stick to the recommended portion sizes, you can slim down without ever slowing down.

For the healthiest, tastiest ingredients, packaged meal

BREAD	CALORIES	FAT	FIBER	CARBS	SODIUM
Arnold Sandwich Thins Seedless Rye	100	1	5	23	210
Arnold Natural Flax & Fiber	110	2	5	21	150
Aunt Millie's Healthy Goodness Fiber & Flavor Potato Bread	120	1.5	3	24	250
Aunt Millie's Healthy Goodness Whole Grain White Bread	95	1.5	5	21	180
Aunt Millie's Fiber for Life Light Five Grain Bread	80	1	5	20	180
Aunt Millie's Hearth Whole Grain Hamburger Buns	140	2	3	27	310
Ener-G Foods Corn Loaf	40	2	3	7	50
Ener-G Foods Seattle Hamburger & Hot Dog Buns	180	6	4	32	210
Ener-G Foods Brown English Muffins with Flax	180	5	4	33	240
Flatout Original Light wraps	90	2.5	9	16	320
Food for Life Ezekiel 4:9 Organic Sprouted 100% Whole Grain Flourless Bread	80	0.5	3	15	75
Food for Life Genesis 1:29 Organic Sprouted Grain & Seed Bread	80	2	3	14	65
Food for Life Organic 7-Sprouted Grains Flourless Bread	80	0.5	3	15	80
Food for Life Organic 7-Sprouted 100% Flourless Sprouted Grain English Muffins	80	1	3	16	120
Food for Life Ezekiel 4:9 Organic Prophet's Pocket Bread	100	0.5	4	21	120
Food for Life Ezekiel 4:9 Organic Sprouted Grain Sesame Burger Buns	170	1.5	6	32	180
French Meadow Sprouted Cinnamon Raisin Bread	100	0.5	3	19	90
French Meadow Sprouted 16 Grain & Seed Bread	110	2.5	4	17	80
French Meadow Sprouted Grain Bread	100	0.5	4	18	85
French Meadow Sprouted 16 Grain & Seed Bagels	250	2.5	10	42	220
French Meadow Sprouted Cinnamon Raisin Bagels	270	1.5	7	50	270
French Meadow Sprouted Grain Tortillas	150	0.5	5	27	160
La Tortilla Factory Whole Wheat 100-Calorie Tortilla Wraps	100	1.5	8	24	320

Nutritional information is per individual portion. Check labels for portion size.

	CALORIES	FAT	FIBER	CARBS	SODIUM
La Tortilla Factory Extra Virgin Olive Oil Tomato Basil SoftWraps	100	3	12	20	360
Storye Classic Rye Bread	145	1	8	44	221
Storye Fine Rye Bread	157	1	6	47	201
Storye Classic Rye Bread with Carrots	155	1	6	46	274
Storye Fine Rye Bread with Fruit and Nuts	170	5	6	43	158
Thomas' 100% Whole Wheat Bagel Thins	110	1	5	24	190
Thomas' 100% Whole Wheat English Muffins	120	1	3	23	220
Thomas' Light Multi-Grain English Muffins	100	1	8	26	180
CEREAL					
Barbara's High Fiber Original	180	1.5	14	42	140
Barbara's High Fiber Flax & Granola	200	3	10	42	140
Barbara's High Fiber Cranberry	190	1.5	10	42	140
Barbara's Shredded Spoonfuls Multigrain	120	1.5	4	24	200
Barbara's Puffins Cinnamon	90	1	6	26	150
Barbara's Puffins Honey Rice	120	1	3	25	80
Barbara's Puffins Multigrain	110	0	3	25	80
Bear Naked 100% Pure & Natural Granola Peak Protein	140	7	3	15	25
Bear Naked 100% Natural Nut Cluster Crunch Honey Almond	180	1.5	3	40	220
Bob's Red Mill Organic High Fiber Hot Cereal	150	5	10	27	0
Bob's Red Mill Gluten Free Quick Rolled Oats	180	3	5	29	0
Cascadian Farm Hearty Morning Cereal	200	3	8	43	360
Cheerios Oat Cluster Crunch	100	1	2	22	135
Fiber One Original Cereal	60	1	14	25	105
Food for Life Ezekiel 4:9 Organic Sprouted 100% Whole Grain Flourless Almond Cereal	200	3	6	38	190

	CALORIES	FAT	FIBER	CARBS	SODIUM
Food for Life Ezekiel 4:9 Organic Sprouted Whole Grain Flourless Golden Flax Cereal	180	2.5	6	37	190
GrandyOats Organic Granola Mainely Maple	200	7	4	31	110
Kashi Good Friends Cereal	160	1.5	12	42	110
Kashi GoLean Cereal	140	1	10	30	85
Kashi GoLean Crisp! Toasted Berry Crumble	180	3.5	8	35	125
Kashi GoLean Crunch! Honey Almond Flax	200	4.5	8	36	140
Kellogg's All-Bran Original Cereal	80	1	10	23	80
Kellogg's Corn Flakes	100	0	1	24	200
Mona's Original Granola	140	7	3	16	0
Nature's Path Optimum Banana Almond	190	6	5	35	140
Nature's Path Optimum Cranberry Ginger	190	2.5	8	41	95
Nature's Path Flax Plus Flakes	110	1.5	5	23	135
Nature's Path Heritage Flakes	120	1	5	24	130
Nature's Path Mesa Sunrise Flakes	120	1	3	24	125
Nature's Path Millet Rice Flakes	120	2	3	22	115
Nature's Path Multigrain Oatbran Flakes	110	1	5	24	110
Nature's Path SmartBran	90	1	13	24	130
Nature's Path Whole O's	110	1.5	3	25	115
Nature's Path Hemp Plus Granola	260	10	5	36	45
Nature's Path Peanut Butter Granola	260	11	4	35	75
Nature's Path Pomegran Plus Granola	250	9	4	38	60
Nature's Path Vanilla Almond Flax Plus Granola	250	9	5	36	80
Nature's Path Agave Plus Granola	250	9	4	37	95
Post Grape-Nuts	200	1	7	48	290
Post Shredded Wheat	160	1	6	37	0
Post Raisin Bran	190	1	8	46	250
CHIPS					
Beanitos Black Bean Chips	140	7	5	15	55
Beanitos Pinto Bean & Flax Chips	140	8	5	15	55
Beanitos Pinto Bean & Flax with Cheddar Cheese Chips	140	8	5	14	140
Beanitos Black Bean with Chipotle BBQ Chips	140	7	5	15	150

	CALORIES	FAT	FIBER	CARBS	SODIUM
Corazonas Lightly Salted Tortilla Chips	140	7	3	18	75
Corazonas Squeeze of Lime Tortilla Chips	140	7	3	17	140
Corazonas Parmesan Peppercorn Potato Chips	140	6	2	18	160
Flatout Garlic Herb Crisps	120	4	5	16	330
Flatout Four Cheese Crisps	130	4.5	5	15	290
Flatout Multigrain Crisps	120	4	5	16	240
Food Should Taste Good Multigrain Chips	140	6	3	18	80
Newman's Own Organics Soy Crisps Barbeque	110	3.5	3	14	390
Newman's Own Organics Soy Crisps Cinnamon Sugar	120	4	3	15	170
Newman's Own Organics Soy Crisps White Cheddar	120	4	3	13	290

CRACKERS

	CALORIES	FAT	FIBER	CARBS	SODIUM
Archer Farms Simply Balanced Snack Crackers: Sun-Dried Tomato & Basil	130	3	2	24	220
Back to Nature Harvest Whole Wheat Crackers	120	4.5	3	19	140
Kashi TLC Pita Crisps Original 7 Grain with Sea Salt	120	3	5	22	180
Kashi TLC Pita Crisps Zesty Salsa	120	3	5	22	180
Triscuit Original Crackers	120	4.5	3	19	180
Triscuit Hint of Salt Crackers	130	5	3	19	50
Triscuit Rosemary & Olive Oil Crackers	120	4	3	20	135
Wasa Thin & Crispy Flatbread Original	70	1.5	1	12	130
Wasa Thin & Crispy Flatbread Sesame	70	2	1	11	100
Wasa Thin & Crispy Flatbread Rosemary	70	1.5	1	12	180
Wasa Fiber Crispbread Crackers	35	0.5	2	8	60
Wheat Thins Fiber Selects	120	4.5	5	22	260

FROZEN FOOD (BREAKFAST)

	CALORIES	FAT	FIBER	CARBS	SODIUM
Amy's Kitchen Breakfast Burrito	270	8	5	38	540
Amy's Kitchen Breakfast Scramble Wrap	380	19	4	30	490
Amy's Kitchen Multi-Grain Hot Cereal Bowl	190	1.5	5	40	300
Amy's Kitchen Steel-Cut Oats Hot Cereal Bowl	220	3.5	5	42	190
Amy's Kitchen Tofu Scramble	320	19	4	19	580
Kellogg's Eggo Nutri-Grain Whole Wheat Waffles	170	6	3	26	400

	CALORIES	FAT	FIBER	CARBS	SODIUM
Kellogg's Eggo Nutri-Grain Blueberry Waffles	180	5	3	31	370
Lean Pockets Applewood Bacon, Egg & Low Fat Cheese	260	9	3	37	510
Smart Ones Breakfast Quesadilla	230	7	7	29	580
Smart Ones Stuffed Breakfast Sandwich	240	7	3	30	570
FROZEN MEALS					
Amy's Kitchen Baked Ziti Bowl	390	12	6	62	590
Amy's Kitchen Brown Rice & Vegetables Bowl, light in sodium	260	9	5	36	270
Amy's Kitchen Mexican Casserole Bowl, light in sodium	370	16	7	48	390
Amy's Kitchen Baked Ziti Kids Meal	360	12	4	57	460
Amy's Kitchen Indian Paneer Tikka	320	19	5	36	550
Amy's Kitchen Indian Mattar Paneer, light in sodium	370	11	6	54	390
Amy's Kitchen Asian Noodle Stir-Fry	300	7	5	50	630
Amy's Kitchen Thai Stir-Fry	310	11	5	45	420
Amy's Kitchen Veggie Loaf Whole Meal, light in sodium	290	8	10	47	340
Amy's Kitchen Light & Lean Spinach Lasagna	250	5	5	40	540
Amy's Kitchen Light & Lean Pasta & Veggies	210	5	3	33	470
Amy's Kitchen Light & Lean Soft Taco Fiesta	220	4.5	5	40	560
Amy's Kitchen Light & Lean Black Bean & Cheese Enchilada	240	4.5	4	44	480
Amy's Kitchen Indian Spinach Tofu Wrap	270	13	6	28	690
Amy's Kitchen Southwestern Burrito	290	10	6	38	680
Amy's Kitchen Chili & Cornbread Whole Meal	340	6	10	59	680
Amy's Kitchen Black Bean Enchilada Whole Meal with Spanish Rice and Beans	330	8	9	53	740
Amy's Kitchen Black Bean Vegetable Enchilada	160	6	4	22	390
Dr. Praeger's Falafel Flats	110	4.5	4	14	135
Dr. Praeger's Burrito Bites	130	3	4	20	210
Dr. Praeger's California Veggie Balls	80	2.5	3	10	190
Ethnic Gourmet Pad Thai with Tofu	420	8	3	73	720
Ethnic Gourmet Lemongrass & Basil Chicken	380	9	5	56	310
Ethnic Gourmet Malay Chicken Curry	410	11	3	59	530
Ethnic Gourmet Chicken Korma	340	9	3	44	720

	CALORIES	FAT	FIBER	CARBS	SODIUM
Evol Cilantro Lime Chicken Burrito	320	7	4	49	450
Evol Veggie Fajita Burrito	290	3.5	5	56	440
Evol Basic Bean & Cheese Burrito	360	7	8	60	620
Evol Tofu & Spinach Sauté Burrito	300	5	6	52	510
Guiltless Gourmet California Veggie Wrap	230	7	6	40	470
Guiltless Gourmet Mediterranean Spinach Wrap	220	6	6	39	410
Guiltless Gourmet Black Bean Chipotle Wrap	230	6	7	47	450
Healthy Choice Oven Roasted Chicken	240	5	4	33	530
Healthy Choice Top Chef Café Steamers Grilled Chicken Pesto with Vegetables	310	9	3	34	550
Healthy Choice Top Chef Café Steamers Chicken Margherita	320	8	4	40	600
Healthy Choice Café Steamers Grilled Basil Chicken	270	6	7	34	600
Healthy Choice Café Steamers Lemon Garlic Chicken and Shrimp	260	6	6	35	600
Healthy Choice Top Chef Café Steamers Grilled Vegetables Mediterranean	230	2.5	7	44	600
Healthy Choice Honey Balsamic Chicken	220	3.5	5	34	540
Kashi Black Bean Mango	340	8	7	58	380
Kashi Chicken Pasta Pomodoro	280	6	6	38	470
Kashi Chicken Florentine	290	9	5	31	550
Kashi Lemongrass Coconut Chicken	300	8	7	38	680
Kashi Mayan Harvest Bake	340	9	8	58	380
Kashi Pesto Pasta Primavera	290	11	7	37	750
Kashi Red Curry Chicken	300	8	6	42	420
Kashi Southwest Style Chicken	310	5	6	49	680
Kashi Sweet & Sour Chicken	320	3.5	6	55	380
Kashi Tuscan Veggie Bake	260	9	8	42	700
Lean Cuisine Sun Dried Tomato Pesto Chicken	270	9	4	28	570
Lean Cuisine Ginger Garlic Stir Fry with Chicken	280	4	5	43	570
Lean Cuisine Salmon with Basil	210	6	5	25	590
Lean Pockets Whole Grain Culinary Creations Grilled Chicken, Mushroom & Wild Rice	250	7	3	39	510

	CALORIES	FAT	FIBER	CARBS	SODIUM
Lean Pockets Whole Grain Turkey, Broccoli & Cheese	260	8	4	38	430
Lean Pockets Whole Grain Culinary Creations Chipotle Chicken	260	7	4	39	530

FROZEN SIDES

	CALORIES	FAT	FIBER	CARBS	SODIUM
Amy's Kitchen Organic Vegetarian Baked Beans	140	0.5	6	28	480
Amy's Kitchen Organic Traditional Refried Beans light in sodium	140	3	6	22	190
Dr. Praeger's Potato Pancakes	100	4	3	13	190
Dr. Praeger's Sweet Potato Pancakes	80	2	3	12	140

HOT CEREAL

	CALORIES	FAT	FIBER	CARBS	SODIUM
Bob's Red Mill 7 Grain Hot Cereal	140	1.5	6	28	0
Country Choice Organic Old Fashioned Oats	150	3	4	27	0
Country Choice Organic Quick Oats	150	3	4	27	0
Country Choice Organic Multigrain Hot Cereal	130	1	5	29	0
Country Choice Organic Steel Cut Oats	150	3	4	27	0
Country Choice Organic Maple Instant Oatmeal	170	2	3	32	60
Country Choice Organic Apple Cinnamon Instant Oatmeal	140	1.5	3	22	60
Country Choice Organic Original with Flax Instant Oatmeal	110	2	3	19	0
Hodgson Mill Multi Grain Hot Cereal with Flaxseed & Soy	160	3	6	25	0
Nature's Path Organic Apple Cinnamon Hot Oatmeal	210	2.5	4	40	100
Nature's Path Organic Flax Plus Hot Oatmeal	210	3	5	38	140
Nature's Path Organic Hemp Plus Hot Oatmeal	160	2.5	4	30	105
Nature's Path Organic Maple Nut Hot Oatmeal	210	4	4	38	100
Nature's Path Organic MultiGrain Raisin Spice Oatmeal	180	1	4	39	100
Nature's Path Organic Optimum Cinnamon, Blueberry, and Flaxseed Oatmeal	150	2.5	3	29	115
Quaker Hearty Medleys Apple Cranberry Almond	130	2.5	3	27	135

MUFFINS

	CALORIES	FAT	FIBER	CARBS	SODIUM
Aunt Millie's Whole Grain Blueberry Muffins	170	8	3	23	150

	CALORIES	FAT	FIBER	CARBS	SODIUM
Aunt Millie's Whole Grain Brownie Muffins	220	9	2	35	130
Fiber One Whole Grain Wild Blueberry & Oats Muffins	170	4	7	33	200
Vitalicious VitaMuffins Deep Chocolate	100	1.5	9	26	140
Vitalicious VitaMuffins CranBran	100	0	5	22	140
Vitalicious VitaMuffins Golden Corn	100	1	6	25	135
Vitalicious VitaMuffins BlueBran	200	0	13	48	330
Vitalicious VitaTops Banana Nut	100	2	8	22	105
Vitalicious VitaTops Apple Crumb	100	1	8	25	105
Vitalicious VitaTops Fudgy Peanut Butter Chip	100	1.5	8	26	150

OTHER

	CALORIES	FAT	FIBER	CARBS	SODIUM
King Arthur Flour Hi-Maize Natural Fiber	15	0	6	9	0
King Arthur Flour Hi-Maize High Fiber Flour	90	0	5	23	0
Annie Chun's Pad Thai Brown Rice Noodles	200	1	4	44	10
Annie Chun's Maifun Brown Rice Noodles	200	1	4	44	10
Archer Farms Simply Balanced Lemon & Pepper Fusilli	240	2	4	48	470
Archer Farms Simply Balanced Red Pepper Penne	250	2	7	49	460
Archer Farms Simply Balanced Cajun Style Beans & Rice Lunch Bowl	250	1	9	51	430
Bumble Bee Sensations Seasoned Lemon & Cracked Pepper Tuna Medley Bowl	110	3	0	2	350
StarKist Charlie's Lunch Kit Chunk Light	210	8	2	19	580

PASTA

	CALORIES	FAT	FIBER	CARBS	SODIUM
Annie's Lower Sodium Mac & Cheese	270	4	2	47	430
Annie's Organic 5-Grain Elbows & White Cheddar	260	4	3	46	570
Annie's Bunny Pasta with Yummy Cheese	260	3.5	3	46	400
Annie's Penne Pasta with Alfredo	220	3.5	2	37	430
Annie's Curly Fettuccine with White Cheddar & Broccoli Sauce	200	2.5	2	37	450
Archer Farms Simply Balanced Whole Wheat Pasta	200	1	4	43	0
Barilla Plus Pasta	210	2	4	38	25

	CALORIES	FAT	FIBER	CARBS	SODIUM
Barilla Whole Grain Pasta	200	1.5	6	41	0
Dreamfields Pasta (spaghetti)	190	1	5	41	10
Racconto Essentials Heart Health 8 Whole Grain Pasta	190	1	7	41	0
Racconto Essentials Glycemic Health 8 Whole Grain Pasta	190	1	11	42	10
Ronzoni Healthy Harvest Whole Grain Penne Rigate	180	1	6	41	0
Ronzoni Healthy Harvest Whole Grain Lasagna	180	1.5	7	39	0
Ronzoni Healthy Harvest Whole Grain Linguine	180	1	6	41	0
Ronzoni Healthy Harvest Whole Grain Rotini	180	1	6	41	0
Ronzoni Healthy Harvest Whole Grain Spaghetti	180	1	6	41	0
Ronzoni Smart Taste Spaghetti	170	0.5	5	40	0

RICE

Near East Whole Grain Blends Brown Rice Pilaf	180	1	3	41	600
Near East Whole Grain Blends Roasted Garlic	190	2	5	41	510
Near East Whole Grain Blends Roasted Pecan and Garlic	220	5	4	38	480
Near East Creative Grains Mix Creamy Parmesan	240	3	3	49	690
Uncle Ben's Whole Grain Boil-in-Bag Brown Rice	170	1.5	2	36	0

SNACKS

Annie's Whole Wheat Cheddar Bunnies	140	6	2	18	250
Annie's Chocolate Bunny Grahams	130	4.5	2	21	75
Annie's Honey Bunny Grahams	140	4.5	2	22	170
Archer Farms Simply Balanced Peach Mango Fruit & Yogurt Bars	90	0.5	2	21	10
Archer Farms Simply Balanced Strawberry Banana Fruit & Yogurt Bars	110	0.5	3	29	0
Archer Farms Simply Balanced Granola Bars: Blueberry Almond Flax	150	3	4	26	40
Baked Lay's potato chips	120	2	2	23	135
Clif Chocolate Chip Crunch Bars	180	8	3	27	100
Clif Honey Oat Crunch Bars	180	8	3	28	110
Clif Peanut Butter Crunch Bars	190	9	3	25	115
Clif White Chocolate Macadamia Nut Crunch Bars	190	9	3	25	115
Evol Mini Burritos Bean & Cheddar	190	3.5	4	32	360

	CALORIES	FAT	FIBER	CARBS	SODIUM
Evol Mini Burritos Veggie Fajita	160	2	3	30	280
Extend Snacks ExtendBar Sugar-Free Chocolate Delight	150	3	6	20	200
Fiber One Chewy Bars Oats & Caramel	140	3.5	9	30	105
Fiber One Chewy Bars Oats & Strawberry with Almonds	140	3	9	29	90
Fiber One Chewy Bars Oats & Peanut Butter	150	4.5	9	28	105
Fiber One Chewy Bars Oats & Chocolate	140	4	9	29	95
Hershey's Kisses Special Dark Mildly Sweet Chocolates	180	12	3	25	15
Kashi TLC Cereal Bars Baked Cherry Vanilla	120	3	3	23	100
Kashi TLC Cereal Bars Blackberry Graham	130	3	3	24	125
Kashi TLC Cereal Bars Ripe Strawberry	130	3	3	24	100
Kashi TLC Chewy Granola Bars Cherry Dark Chocolate	120	2	4	24	65
Kashi TLC Chewy Granola Bars Honey Almond Flax	140	5	4	19	105
Kashi TLC Chewy Granola Bars Peanut Peanut Butter	140	5	4	19	85
Kashi TLC Chewy Granola Bars Trail Mix	140	5	4	20	95
Kashi TLC Peanutty Dark Chocolate Layered Granola Bars	130	4.5	4	20	80
Kashi TLC Crunchy Granola Bars Pumpkin Spice Flax	170	6	4	25	135
Kashi TLC Crunchy Granola Bars Honey Toasted 7-Grain	170	5	4	26	150
Kashi GoLean Crunchy! Chocolate Almond Protein & Fiber Bars	170	5	5	27	210
Kashi GoLean Crunchy! Chocolate Pretzel Protein & Fiber Bars	160	3	5	28	250
Kashi GoLean Crunchy! Chocolate Caramel Protein & Fiber Bars	150	3	6	28	220
Kashi TLC Cookies Oatmeal Raisin Flax	130	4.5	4	20	70
Kashi TLC Cookies Happy Trail Mix	140	5	4	21	75
Kashi TLC Cookies Oatmeal Dark Chocolate	130	5	4	20	65
Kellogg's FiberPlus Antioxidants Dark Chocolate Almond Bars	130	5	9	24	50
Kellogg's FiberPlus Antioxidants Chocolate Chip Bars	120	4	9	26	55
Kellogg's FiberPlus Antioxidants Chocolatey Peanut Butter Bars	130	5	9	24	95
Kind Cranberry Almond + Antioxidants snack bars	190	13	3	20	20
Kind Peanut Butter Dark Chocolate + Protein snack bars	200	13	3	17	50

	CALORIES	FAT	FIBER	CARBS	SODIUM
Kind Blueberry Pecan + Fiber snack bars	180	10	5	23	25
Lärabar Cherry Pie mini bar	90	4	2	14	0
Laughing Cow Mini Babybel Cheddar cheese	70	5	0	0	140
Laughing Cow Mini Babybel Original cheese	70	6	0	0	170
Laughing Cow Mini Babybel Bonbel cheese	70	6	0	0	170
Laughing Cow Mini Babybel Gouda cheese	80	6	0	0	170
Laughing Cow Mini Babybel Light cheese	50	3	0	0	160
Laughing Cow Light Creamy Swiss wedges	35	1.5	0	1	210
Laughing Cow Light Garlic & Herb wedges	35	1.5	0	1	210
Laughing Cow Light French Onion wedges	35	1.5	0	1	210
Laughing Cow Light Blue Cheese wedges	35	1.5	0	2	230
Luna Protein Chocolate Peanut Butter bars	190	9	3	20	220
Luna Protein Cookie Dough bars	180	6	3	21	230
Luna Protein Chocolate Cherry Bar Almond	180	6	3	21	115
Nature's Path Organic Sunny Hemp Granola Bars	140	3.5	3	24	90
Nature Valley Sweet & Salty Nut Almond Granola Bars	160	7	2	22	150
Nature Valley Fruit & Nut Trail Mix Bars	140	4	2	25	65
Nature Valley Peanut Butter Crunchy Granola Bars	190	7	2	28	180
Nature Valley Oats 'n Honey Crunchy Granola Bars	190	6	2	29	160
Newman's Own Organics Spelt Pretzels	120	1	4	23	240
Newman's Own Organics Hi-Protein Pretzels	120	1.5	4	22	230
Newman's Own Organics Thin Stick Pretzels	110	1.5	4	22	180
Newman's Own Organics Dried Apricots	110	0	2	25	0
Newman's Own Organics Dried Apple Rings	120	0	2	29	0
Nutri-Grain Blueberry Cereal Bars	120	3	3	24	110
Odwalla Banana Nut Bars	220	5	5	39	105
Odwalla Blueberry Swirl Bars	200	3	4	41	125
Quaker Fiber & Omega-3 Peanut Butter Chocolate Granola Bars	150	5	9	25	35
Quaker Oatmeal to Go High Fiber Maple Brown Sugar	210	4	10	43	230
Sabra Classic Single Serve Hummus	150	11	3	9	260

	CALORIES	FAT	FIBER	CARBS	SODIUM
SOUP					
Amy's Kitchen Organic Lentil	180	5	6	25	590
Amy's Kitchen Organic Lentil Vegetable, light in sodium	160	4	8	24	340
Amy's Kitchen Organic Lentil, light in sodium	180	5	6	25	290
Amy's Kitchen Organic Medium Chili with Vegetables	230	6	9	34	590
Amy's Kitchen Organic Medium Chili, light in sodium	280	9	7	35	340
Amy's Kitchen Organic Spicy Chili, light in sodium	280	9	7	35	340
Campbell's Chunky Healthy Request Vegetable	120	1	4	24	410
Campbell's Select Harvest Chicken Tuscany	90	1.5	4	12	650
Campbell's Select Harvest Light Roasted Chicken with Italian Herbs	80	2.5	3	9	650
Pacific Natural Foods Organic Light Sodium Butternut Squash	90	2	3	17	280
Progresso High Fiber Homestyle Minestrone	110	2	7	24	690
Progresso High Fiber Creamy Tomato Basil	130	4	7	26	690
Progresso High Fiber Hearty Vegetable and Noodles	90	1.5	7	18	690
Progresso High Fiber Three-Bean Chili with Beef	140	4	7	23	480
Progresso High Fiber Chicken Tuscany	130	3	7	20	690
VEGGIE BURGERS					
Boca Veggie Patties: Bruschetta Tomato Basil Parmesan	90	1.5	5	9	440
Boca Original Vegan Meatless Burgers	70	0.5	4	6	280
Dr. Praeger's California Veggie Burgers	110	5	4	13	250
Dr. Praeger's Italian Veggie Burgers	110	5	5	13	250
Dr. Praeger's Tex Mex Veggie Burgers	110	4.5	5	13	250
YOGURT					
Chobani Non-Fat Plain Greek Yogurt (6 oz)	100	0	0	7	80
Dannon Activia Peach & Cereal Fiber Yogurt (4 oz)	110	2	3	20	60
Fage Total 0% Plain Greek Yogurt (6 oz)	100	0	0	7	65
Stonyfield Oikos Organic Plain Greek Yogurt (5.3 oz)	80	0	0	6	60
Yoplait Fiber One Yogurt (all flavors) (4 oz)	50	0	5	13	55

Metric Equivalents

The recipes that appear in this cookbook use the standard U.S. method for measuring liquid and dry or solid ingredients (teaspoons, tablespoons, and cups). The information in the following charts is provided to help cooks outside the United States successfully use these recipes. All equivalents are approximate.

Metric Equivalents for Different Types of Ingredients

A standard cup measure of a dry or solid ingredient will vary in weight depending on the type of ingredient. A standard cup of liquid is the same volume for any type of liquid. Use the following chart when converting standard cup measures to grams (weight) or milliliters (volume).

Standard Cup	Fine Powder (e.g., flour)	Grain (e.g., rice)	Granular (e.g., sugar)	Liquid Solids (e.g., butter)	Liquid (e.g., milk)
1	140g	150g	190g	200g	240 ml
¾	105g	113g	143g	150g	180 ml
⅔	93g	100g	125g	133g	160 ml
½	70g	75g	95g	100g	120 ml
⅓	47g	50g	63g	67g	80 ml
¼	35g	38g	48g	50g	60 ml
⅛	18g	19g	24g	25g	30 ml

Useful Equivalents for Liquid Ingredients by Volume

¼ tsp						=	1 ml	
½ tsp						=	2 ml	
1 tsp						=	5 ml	
3 tsp	=	1 Tbsp			=	½ fl oz	=	15 ml
		2 Tbsp	=	⅛ cup	=	1 fl oz	=	30 ml
		4 Tbsp	=	¼ cup	=	2 fl oz	=	60 ml
		5⅓ Tbsp	=	⅓ cup	=	3 fl oz	=	80 ml
		8 Tbsp	=	½ cup	=	4 fl oz	=	120 ml
		10⅔ Tbsp	=	⅔ cup	=	5 fl oz	=	160 ml
		12 Tbsp	=	¾ cup	=	6 fl oz	=	180 ml
		16 Tbsp	=	1 cup	=	8 fl oz	=	240 ml
		1 pt	=	2 cups	=	16 fl oz	=	480 ml
		1 qt	=	4 cups	=	32 fl oz	=	960 ml
						33 fl oz	=	1,000 ml

Useful Equivalents for Dry Ingredients by Weight

(To convert ounces to grams, multiply the number of ounces by 30.)

1 oz	=	¹⁄₁₆ lb	=	30g
4 oz	=	¼ lb	=	120g
8 oz	=	½ lb	=	240g
12 oz	=	¾ lb	=	360g
16 oz	=	1 lb	=	480g

Useful Equivalents for Length

(To convert inches to centimeters, multiply the number of inches by 2.5.)

1 in					=	2.5 cm	
6 in	=	½ ft			=	15 cm	
12 in	=	1 ft			=	30 cm	
36 in	=	3 ft	=	1 yd	=	90 cm	
40 in					=	100 cm	= 1 m

Useful Equivalents for Cooking/Oven Temperatures

	Fahrenheit	Celsius	Gas Mark
Freeze water	32° F	0° C	
Room temperature	68°F	20°C	
Boil water	212°F	100°C	
Bake	325°F	160°C	3
	350°F	180°C	4
	375°F	190°C	5
	400°F	200°C	6
	425°F	220°C	7
	450°F	230°C	8
Broil			Grill

Recipe Index

333

SUBJECT INDEX

Oxmoor House
VP, Publishing
Jim Childs

Editorial Director
Susan Payne Dobbs

Creative Director
Felicity Keane

Brand Manager
Vanessa Tiongson

Managing Editor
Laurie S. Herr

Project Editor
Holly D. Smith

Production Manager
Sue Chodakiewicz

Time Home Entertainment Inc.
Publisher
Richard Fraiman

VP, Strategy &
Business Development
Steven Sandonato

Executive Director,
Marketing Services
Carol Pittard

Executive Director,
Retail & Special Sales
Tom Mifsud

Executive Director,
New Product Development
Peter Harper

Director, Bookazine
Development & Marketing
Laura Adam

Publishing Director
Joy Butts

Finance Director
Glenn Buonocore

Assistant General Counsel
Helen Wan

To order additional publications,
call 800-765-6400
or 800-491-0551

For more books to enrich your
life, visit oxmoorhouse.com. To
search, savor, and share thousands
of recipes, visit myrecipes.com.

Credits
Cover and main photography by **Andrew McCaul**
Food styling by **Stephana Bottom**
Prop styling by **Alistair Turnbull for Pat Bates**

p. 39, 45, 73, 75, 91, 99, 103, 107, 129, 133, 139, 153,
189, Melissa Punch

Chefs p. 260 Puck, ABC via Getty Images; Fieri,
Contour by Getty Images; Cora & Chiarello, Getty Images
p. 262 Fieri, Sherrie Blondin
p. 263 Pasta shells, Con Poulos
p. 264 Puck, Amanda Marsalis
p. 265 BBQ pizza, Kate Sears
p. 266 Cora, David Carlson
p. 267 Sushi, Melissa Punch
p. 268 Hall, Matthew Lyons
p. 269 Chicken mole, Quentin Bacon
p. 270 Chiarello, Frankie Frankeny
p. 271 Fusilli, Kate Sears
p. 272 Arpaia, Courtesy of Donatella Arpaia
p. 273 Crostini, Joseph De Leo
p. 274 Luchetti, Jeff Gleason
p. 275 Rice pudding, Melissa Punch
p. 276 Kumai, Quentin Bacon
p. 277 Barley, Quentin Bacon
p. 278 Ferrare, Todd Porter & Diane Cu
p. 279 Polenta, Andrew McCaul
p. 280 Bastianich, Greg Gayne
p. 281 Scoglio, Andrew McCaul
p. 283 Simmons, Tina Rupp
p. 285 Pizza, Andrew McCaul
p. 286 Torey, John Kernick
p. 287 Cupcakes, Melissa Punch
p. 289 Lewis & Poliafito, Gregg Delman
p. 291 Cookies, Andrew McCaul

Cover: Pasta Primavera, page 112
Back Cover: Top, Oat and Honey Pancakes
with Strawberry Syrup, page 34;
below, Barbecue Chicken Pizza, page 264

Finally, a diet that really works!

Look for even more great *CarbLovers* products to help you shed pounds—while eating your favorite foods!

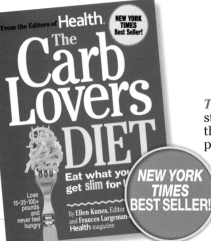

The CarbLovers Diet is the book that started a weight-loss revolution, inspiring thousands of women to drop all the pounds they wanted without ever feeling hungry! Filled with hundreds of tips, expert advice, delicious recipes, and real-life success stories, it's the diet book you'll turn to again and again.

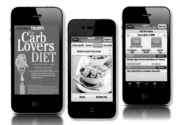

The New *CarbLovers* App for iPhone® is a vital tool to help you get and stay slim! Now you can have instant access to *CarbLovers* meal plans, recipes, and expert advice. Tap yourself slim with a weight-loss tracker and a handy on-the-go meal guide! Available on iTunes.

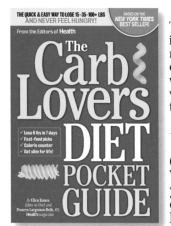

The *CarbLovers Diet Pocket Guide* is the perfect pocket-size companion resource for those looking for quick and easy on-the-go *CarbLovers* insight. It will help you eat what you love and lose weight by showing you how to choose the right foods no matter where you are.

Get Slim Now!
Visit carblovers.com and order your copies today. Become a fan of *CarbLovers* on Facebook. Follow @Carbloversdiet on Twitter.